WHAT IS THAT

LIGHT

AT THE END OF THE

TUNNEL?

Living with Cone Rod Dystrophy and loving life!

VIDA BYAS

ISBN: 1478213914
ISBN-13: 9781478213918

If I left out any source on my resource list, please contact me at: vida.byas@yahoo.com

ACKNOWLEDGEMENT

When all in my world began to fade
And I could no longer see the color of my face
I grew my thoughts and words in shade
And learned to live in my new place.
I hope this book is of comfort to every reader. It is dedicated to my
loved ones and to all who are living with disabilities and loving life.

V. Byas

CONTENTS

FOREWORD

I was born in the Dominican Republic. I am descended from Caribbeans who migrated to the Dominican Republic during the nineteenth century. The émigrés to my hometown of San Pedro de Macoris came mainly from the British Virgin Islands and other islands in the Upper and Lesser Antilles. These people came from Tortola, St. Kitts, St. Christopher, Nevis, Antigua Montserrat, and other islands. These people left behind all they had ever known for the chance of having a brighter future. They risked going to the Dominican Republic, a place of completely unknown cultures, customs, and languages, in search of work. Upon arriving in the Dominican Republic, the immigrants were not readily accepted. However, they brought a distinctly British and exceptionally stoic view of life. Notably, they had a very strong work ethic and a reverence for education.

Most jobs were closed to them, so they worked primarily in the sugarcane fields, sugar mills, and on the docks. Another avenue that opened for them was in the very new and favorite past time sweeping the island—baseball. Descendants of these immigrants are predominant in Dominican baseball leagues as well as in the United States major leagues. Over time, these immigrants assimilated and integrated into Dominican culture. They made gains in the area of education, agriculture, and entrepreneurship. They established social mediums such as societies, lodges, and schools. Today in the Dominican Republic, many traditions, foods, language assimilations, and religious and cultural views can be directly attributed to the contributions made by these communities.

Everywhere around the world, words are used to describe and characterize groups and peoples, and these can be both positive and negative in nature. These descriptors can be chosen by a people to reflect what is important for them to convey to others, but more often, words are externally applied to reflect the perceptions of others. The words and context used are relative to the community in question and can be a matter of correct or incorrect perceptions, worldviews, or customs.

Dominicans were wary of the new immigrants who came from so many different islands. Ultimately, they accepted these people into their society and Dominicans began to attach certain attributes to the entire migratory group. Among these attributes was the perception that these islanders were strict, stoic, and unbending in their views. They were noted to have high intellectual abilities and a capacity for doing just about anything to make money. They were seen as people who were very religious with high integrity, and as having a no-nonsense demeanor. They were also predominantly of African descent.

Gradually, the term Cocolo or Cocola was used to refer to a person specifically of African descent and from any of these islands. Many such communities settled in towns everywhere in the Dominican Republic, but particularly on the southeastern coast where they had access to docks and great concentrations of sugarcane fields and sugar mills. Large populations grew. During the colonial period, my hometown of San Pedro de Macoris was an important coastal town that bustled with energy around the docks. It is easy to see why so many Cocolos settled there. As they were not allowed to construct their houses within the town limits, they built their homes on the outskirts and less attractive areas of the town. These outlying areas today are notable for the generations of Cocolo families that continue to live there. My family is one of them.

My father, an educator who ultimately became a regional governor, once wrote a self-published treatise regarding the origin of the word

Cocolo. Largely unread popularly, but of great pride in our family, he argued that one theory could be that the word was a perversion of the word Tortola. It is true that the largest immigrant population came from the capital of the British colonies in the Virgin Islands, Tortola. He argued that native Dominicans of the time, a mixed people of Spanish, Taino Indian, and African cultures, could not understand or say the words that they heard these people use to describe themselves. The immigrants had British and Creole accents, vocabulary, and intonation patterns alien to the Dominicans. In his treatment of his argument, we can readily believe that the native Dominicans had trouble understanding them. My father believed that Totolos (later becoming Cocolos) could have been an easy and Spanish-sounding word to be applied to everyone who came from these islands.

My maternal grandfather was a Tortolian, and my paternal grandfather was from St. Kitts. Just as in their "old world," these immigrant families were paternalistic in nature. This view fit in quite well with Dominican society, which also places the father at the top of the family. It is from my paternal grandfather that the most prominent traits, views, and cultural mores stem from that I see in my family and myself. My grandmother also had a great impact on how the women in our family behave and think. Her family came from St. Christopher, and the women had very definite ideas about what it was to be a woman. They saw themselves as equal partners, even as they navigated this paternalistic society with diplomatic aplomb and natural instinct. I have carried over to my own children this curious mixture of Dominican and Cocolian traits, culture, customs, and traditions.

Growing up Cocola, I heard many traditional sayings from the Cocolo cultural experience vault. Some reflected their deep religious convictions, and others their cultural and life experiences. One saying that I often heard from my grandmother was, "We always have a plate full of trouble but now we have a pot full," or some such variation on that theme. Our elders wanted us, the children, to learn a profound lesson about our humanity. Life is always challenging us with situations that we learn to manage and to solve.

Occasionally, life throws us for a loop. We are blindsided by an event so overwhelming that it requires all of our strength, will, and resources to overcome. Sometimes we even wonder if we can make it. The Cocolo viewpoint is that an individual can overcome any difficulty if that person brings all internal and external resources possible to the challenge. A Cocolo is expected to come out on the other side stronger and more resilient than before. Thus, the Cocolo parent's advice to the young child is, "When you have a pot full of trouble, best to pick up a spoon and start digging until you see the bottom." This part of the Cocolo philosophy.

Cone Rod Dystrophy was such a life-changing event for me. It was overwhelming to know that I had a condition, which, over time would cause me to go blind. Most of us view our eyes as the first and most important of all our senses. It allows us to interact with the world in meaningful ways. We depend on our eyes for clues to events, emotions, physical states, and the completion of all kinds of tasks in our lives. Even more so, the thought of not being able to see the dear faces of your loved ones and those yet to be born into your family can be disheartening. The eyes have found a prominent place in most aspects of human and cultural life. Even the most common sayings often allude to the eyes: Beauty is in the eyes of the beholder, and the eyes are the window to the soul. These are testimony to how important vision is to us. Even minimal visual changes can be very frightening, traumatic, and cause a person to suffer anxiety. For many, as it was for me initially, the prospect of blindness is a devastating diagnosis.

Millions of people in the United States, and many more in greater numbers worldwide, must deal with profound changes in their eyesight. An ever-growing number of these individuals will be diagnosed with a retinal problem, such as the genetically linked Cone Rod Dystrophy. For me, the key to understanding, managing, and adjusting to blindness began with a series of intellectual and analytical activities.

Cone Rod Dystrophy patients recognizes a change of some sort to their vision. At the onset, it may not register with the patient that this is a life-altering event. Many factors can affect the eyesight. These may include diet, illness that can be controlled with the appropriate treatment, or medications. The patient visits the doctor to consult with a professional who can shed some light on what could be wrong. Optimism and hope is present, and generally, anxiety is not something that is profoundly felt at first. The eye professional typically conducts or orders a series of screenings to determine the cause of the vision change—a journey that will eventually lead to the discovery of the potential cause of the problem and hopefully a diagnosis. What ensues is a long process culminating in steps that will help the patient transition from a sighted person to one who is visually impaired. Arriving at this stage of the process is overwhelming enough; going forward into a new way of life is a challenge of gladiatorial proportions, and it means coming into a new way of being.

Each of these steps requires a knowledge base, manipulation of the gathered information, and practical real-life applications. One learns to manage each step of the condition in ways that make sense and allow for hope, positivity, and productivity. When one is going blind, it is normal to feel at a loss, alienated, and more dependent on others. Until one can learn more about the condition that is leading to the blindness, the treatments available, strategies and tools that can be utilized, and new skills for coping with the vision loss, these feelings of helplessness and hopelessness have the power to take over your life. Once we have discovered how to manage the situation, we gradually become more empowered.

By educating myself about Cone Rod Dystrophy, finding out how to manage the effects of the condition, and learning new skills and strategies for facing the new challenges, I discovered that these formed the basis for discovering inner strength, courage, and determination to continue loving life as a blind individual.

Each degree of vision loss that I experience is a gain in knowledge of how to solve, or better said, how to unravel the new challenges posed. I figure out new ways to complete the various tasks of everyday living. I surprise myself constantly when I discover what I can achieve, and my days are often filled with whimsical laughter at the gaffs I make. As someone once wisely said, if you can keep your head when all around you others are losing theirs, you can be successful in your endeavor and happy, too.

Becoming blind due to Cone Rod Dystrophy compels you to learn a new state of being, just as any other life condition, trait, illness, or circumstance will do. It becomes a normal part of who you are and the way you do things in life, similar to what is experienced by individuals living with cancer, paralysis, mental health issues, and learning disabilities.

One of the most important lessons I have learned throughout this discovery portion of my life is to look on this condition as another extension of who I am. Being blind is no more and no less than the color of my eyes, my ever-present smile, or the skills I have acquired as a case manager in the area of social services and teaching.

As my life's journey would have it, I am a mother, daughter, sister, friend, lover, and blind. All of these are part of being me. Thus, I am devoted to learning what I can do to meet the challenges and opportunities that lie before me. The more challenging the task, the more dedicated I am to succeed. I have learned that I can rely on my own inner resources and skills to face the challenges that inevitably arise; yet, I am not afraid to ask for external assistance when necessary. After all, this is what everyone has to do to get along in life. I've learned to go about living and loving my life in blindness.

This is my story of blindness dedicated to blind and visually impaired individuals everywhere, particularly those living with Cone Rod Dystrophy. My intent is to help impart basic information to these individuals and their families, colleagues, and friends in order for them to begin their own research. This book offers ways to cope with the condition through seeking the appropriate medical personnel, testing instruments, current treatment strategies, and support systems, and it offers tips on daily living.

This book also helps to shed some basic light on the government programs that may be helpful to the blind and the visually impaired, some honest reflection on the doctor-patient relationship, and finally, some resources to look into for those with the condition.

My attempt is to demonstrate that going blind is a journey of discovery full of challenges and practical solutions. There is no end and no beginning in my mind. Being blind is, astonishingly, just simply my state of being. Over time, I have come to relish the steps I have accomplished that have moved me forward. As my Cone Rod Dystrophy progresses, I look forward to learning how to live as happily as it is possible for any human being to live while managing the vagaries of life. It is my sincere hope that this account of an illumined journey into blindness due to Cone Rod Dystrophy will help light a path for others.

Thank you for sharing my story.

V. Byas

CHAPTER 1:
INTRODUCTION

Revealing family links

Have you been to the doctor lately? Hopefully, you have health insurance or access to health programs. At some point, you will have a conversation with the doctor or other staff members, which may go something like this: "Has anybody in your family had cancer, respiratory illnesses, and blood disorders?" My typical reaction is always, "Not that I am aware of," or "Well, truthfully, doctor, I don't really know."

One of the tools that doctors have at their disposal is a patient's family medical history. This helps them to understand what is ailing the patient, and aids the doctor in the screening process and in achieving a diagnosis. This is an important tool because it will shed light on what kinds of medical conditions exist in your family, and thus what you have probably inherited.

Until I started to deal with the condition I have, Cone Rod Dystrophy, I took this element of the doctor-patient relationship for granted. Probably just like you, I answered the questions that were asked without much thought. As I was to find out eventually, I should have been paying more attention.

The first step in my journey into blindness was to learn all I could about pre-existing eye conditions and illnesses that family members had on both sides of my family. In fact, when I had the opportunity to be seen at the National Institutes of Health, I had to learn about prevalent conditions within my cultural group. This is quite daunting when most of us come from multiple cultural groups, developed or under-developed countries, and have multiple ethnicities. Yet, the work has to begin somewhere; in my case, I had to unravel the mystery of how I came to be blind.

The summer of 1990, my children and I went to the Dominican Republic on our annual visit. Every summer vacation since they were old enough to travel by airplane, we had spent on my home island. I was born in the Dominican Republic, a sun drenched tropical island perhaps two to three hours from the US shore. I think island life is as close to perfect as anything can be. My motto is, "Abraza la vida en el caribe y la vida te besara con fragantes y suaves brisas tropicales." Translation: Embrace life in the Caribbean and life will kiss you back with gentle, fragrant tropical breezes.

In terms of quality of life, it is eons away from the standard in the United States. In 1990, our island was considered a third world country. We still did not have electricity and running water in many parts of the country. Our economy was still largely agricultural based, and we owed more money abroad than we could ever generate. Our people were largely illiterate and lived in utter poverty. I did not know all of this until I arrived in the United States sponsored by my mother, who had left the island in the employment of a diplomatic family in the latter part of the 1960s. I had to learn how poor my home country was from books in the United States. Back on the island, we lived a life that was filled with work, school, church, and enjoying time spent with friends and family. When we were hungry, we found food to eat. If we did not have it at home, the neighbors would share what they had. When we had plenty, we would share ours with them. My grandmother raised chickens, and there were always vegetables to eat. The corner market would let you buy the foodstuff you could not grow and put it on your account.

It was understood that upon arriving in the Dominican Republic for our annual vacation, and even before we went to see my father or any other family members, we would stop and pay our respect to my maternal grandmother and my aunt. It is a tradition that lives on today in the Dominican Republic. Not to comply with this tradition is a grave breach of decorum. Those who don't follow this practice may never live down the fact that they disrespected their elders. I have known friends who found it difficult to go back home again as they were not accepted back in the familial bosom until the breach was healed.

My grandmother and aunt lived on the outskirts of town. The roads to the house where I had been raised until I was twelve years old were unpaved. The dust always rose off the road, blown by the breeze coming from the sea under the blazing sun. The houses were just as I remembered—mostly wooden structures with zinc roofs in the styles reminiscent of the colonial past. Some houses were built high up on concrete foundations, with a balcony or terraza facing the street. Others were built at ground level with tall front doors. Newer houses made of brick or stone were dispersed among them in a mixture of the old and new way of living in one of the oldest barrios in my hometown. As the sun goes down, the older people bring out their chairs and rockers to sit out front and gossip, catch the afternoon breeze, and socialize with passersby.

There were older houses that had been part of the barrio for many generations, but scattered among them were newer houses built by people who had recently come to settle in the area. There were even shanties still standing after being pounded time and again by tropical storms and hurricanes. It was a true neighborhood and a part of my hometown that seemed to have been forgotten by time. People still hauled water from wells and lit the darkness with kerosene lamps. They cooked on grates and still went to the corner grocery store for the daily ingredients for each meal. Whenever I visited as an adult, it was just as untouched as when I was a little girl.

Young people can still be seen taking the afternoon stroll bound for the malecon, the boardwalks by the seashore. Just as in most small towns anywhere, this is the time for getting together with friends and catching up on what is happening in everyone's lives. It is a simple life that has remained unchanged for generations.

As soon as we arrived in 1990, neighbors from every part of our barrio came to greet us as if we had not been there the previous summer. My children and I first went to visit my maternal grandmother, Dulcina, and ask for her blessing in the way that Dominican children have been taught to do. "Bendicion abuela," we would say, and then wait for the blessing that would always come from her. My grandmother raised her head from where she was sitting in her favorite rocker with a homemade quilt on her knees and gave us her blessing, "Dios te bendiga."

My daughter went to her, stroked her gaunt, though amazingly wrinkle-free cheeks (she was ninety-four years of age), and said, "Tantan (which is what we all called her), can you see my hand today?" My grandmother laugh and said, "No child but come and comb my hair; I can feel that."

My grandmother's eyesight, like that of many women in my mother's family, had diminished as she aged. By the time she was seventy, she had completely lost her sight. It has never been determined whether the cause of her blindness was glaucoma, cataracts, diabetes related, or a retinal problem. What seems clear to me now is that all of these ailments are present in my family and seem to occur primarily in the females.

My mother's family originally migrated from St. Christopher and St. Kitts. My great grandmother, Mary Elizabeth, went to the Dominican Republic to look for work; she had been born on a plantation where her mother had been from a slave family. She was a product of a liaison between her mother and the owner of the plantation. As a young woman, Mary left St. Christopher with countless other islanders, enticed by the Spanish landowners who were looking for workers for the cane fields.

This spirit of adventure and the ability to look for opportunities in different shores is a hallmark of the history of my family.

As a young woman working in the fields and living in what were called Bateyes, or sugarcane shantytowns, Mary met and married William. He had come to the island alone from St. Kitts to work in the sugarcane fields as well. Mary, as far as I know, never lost her sight completely as her daughter, Tantan, did years later.

Life in the sugarcane fields was not easy. My grandmother tells me that it was back breaking work that lasted all day throughout the growing season. Workers lived in shanties around the fields and the sugar mill. There were many accidents caused by using the machete. This agricultural tool was ideal for cutting sugarcane and other agricultural products. The field-cutting seasons also included the harvesting of tobacco, pineapples, and coffee. Unfortunately, this tool was also used as a weapon. As my grandmother recalls, the sugar mill towns were rough places. The long, grueling hours under the hot sun created hardships, as did the disagreements and occasional fighting that would break out. In spite of these conditions, sugar mill towns became orderly places in which to work, live, educate, and grow families. Only the very hardy could endure and survive the hardships of this way of life. My family endured, and Mary gave birth to her children there.

Mary and Willie Martin had five children and three were lost in infancy. Out of the living five, one son died at a young age after falling out of a coconut tree. He was their only son, and the couple was hit hard by his death. The remaining four girls all lived to their eighties and nineties, and two died completely blind.

I often asked my grandmother, "Tantan, when did you first notice you were going blind?" and she would say, "When I could no longer knit the blankets for the newborns."

I remembered that she had been able to knit my son a newborn blanket upon his birth in 1981, but by 1984, when my daughter was born, she could no longer see to knit a blanket for her. One of the great tragedies of this is that if she had had access to better health care, vision rehabilitation services, and services for the disabled, she could have continued happily knitting blankets. Not being able to have an heirloom from my grandmother to give my daughter is an acute loss. I often wish I had learned to knit like my grandmother when she had tried to teach me. It was a tradition worth keeping, the handing down of an heirloom despite the reality of blindness.

My grandmother had five children. All of them were born and raised in the sugar mill towns. When automation came to the Dominican Republic and the sugar companies no longer needed many workers to clear sugarcane fields, the sugar mill towns died out one after the other. My grandmother has told me about the difficulty of simply feeding her large family. Many were the days that they did not have anything at all to eat, and if not for the charity of others, they would have been very badly off.

The years of the dictatorship of Rafael Trujillo Molina were characterized in my mother's family as being particularly difficult for Cocolo immigrants. According to their accounts, the dictatorship concentrated on industrializing the country. Many of the agriculturally based jobs requiring masses of people dried up. New job opportunities in tourism, manufacturing, and other skilled areas surfaced. However, the lack education and skills for these jobs successfully stymied the potential for growth of this population. In addition, other factors, such as discriminatory practices and the lack of training and apprenticeship opportunities, helped push more members of these groups into harsher poverty. The years following the collapse of the dictatorship awakened a new fervor for exposing many adversarial and detrimental conditions that Dominicans suffered. Social injustice, poverty, discrimination, and the lack of adequate health care and education were among the social ills that the majority of Dominicans lived under. The government's answer to the loss of certain job sectors, such as sugarcane field and sugar mill work, was the establishment of so called zonas francas, or tax free zones open for investment by foreign individuals and corporations.

By creating an environment favorable to businesses by way of reducing their production costs and tax liabilities, the country attracted investors, and as a byproduct, found another source of revenue—tourism. Attracting these investors did create and provide needed jobs for many, and Dominicans who found jobs in the zona, working for these international businesses from Asia, the Americas, Europe, and other countries, counted themselves lucky. Most Dominicans earned as little as twenty cents and as much as two dollars per day. However, in a country where the majority of people were illiterate, this was a welcome circumstance.

In the Dominican Republic, as well as in many under developed and developing countries, the zona provides substandard job opportunities, but the jobs are there. International companies and of course unscrupulous individuals are able to set up businesses in the Dominican Republic and produce goods largely for export for very little manufacturing or labor costs. These companies manufacture quick and cheap goods for external consumption while exploiting cheap labor.

While travelling back from the Dominican Republic in 2011, I happened to be standing in the security checkpoint at Miami International Airport behind two men. The line was slow, and to pass the time, they were discussing the purpose of their trip to the island. I took notice of the conversation when I heard one man tell the other how easy and lucrative it was to set up business there. He told the other fellow, "You can pay your workers whatever you want, make them work in whatever conditions you want to set up, and no one will say anything." The implication was obvious: poor working conditions, sweatshops, and below-poverty pay are accepted practices. Even under such appalling conditions, zona francas thrive in the Dominican Republic today.

I often wonder if the lean years in my family's history affected our physical makeup in genetically predisposing future generations for years to come. Research studies in underdeveloped and developing countries points to malnutrition and other detrimental factors such as organism mutations as catalysts in causing genetic disorders. The lack of good nutrition and the very elemental effects of poverty create real genetic malfunctions and can cause severe medical issues. The Dominican diet for my ancestors was the same as it is today. The Dominican diet consists of staples such as rice, beans, plantains, yucca, potato, fish, beef, and chicken. This diet is generally adequate and mostly nutritional, but when great majorities of people live perpetually substandard, poverty-stricken lives, they may be genetically or medically predisposed to certain illnesses and conditions. Living in extreme poverty is much more than going through some "lean times." It is living for long periods in "bread and sugar-water times," as my grandmother called them, because that is all there is to eat.

Out of the five children she had, my uncle Alfredo developed diabetes, which eventually killed him. Two of my aunts and my mother all have diabetes, and two of my aunts have glaucoma. Whether any of the women in my mother's family had Cone Rod Deficiency or any other retinal impairment is unknown. These women never had the opportunity to go to eye doctors early on. In the case of my grandmother, by the time my family had enough money to take her to an eye specialist, she had already developed cataracts. One of the key elements in tracing the development of my eye condition has been my knowledge of my family's medical history. In particular, it has been interesting to note that just like many of the women in my family I too have the propensity for developing glaucoma. My eye specialists have told me that my inner eye shape is prevalent among those who develop this disease.

In addition, I too have developed cataracts, as many other women in my family have. These are not coincidences; they are strong correlations. It is possible that many of the diagnoses these women received were in error. Could it be that the symptoms they were reporting stemmed from retinal disorders? What is known is that eye conditions can be easily misdiagnosed. It is only through various eye tests done by specialists that a conclusive diagnosis can be made.

On that summer in 1990, while visiting with my family, I asked my grandmother what she could see. Her response was that she saw the light. I never understood that until years later when I too started to lose my vision.

My mother says I was born premature because she did not know she was pregnant. She never had prenatal care, and she says that she only knew she was having a baby when my birth began—when she was only six and a half months pregnant! She often wonders if it is her fault that I am now going blind. As a newborn, those who knew me thought I would not live to celebrate my first birthday. My people were determined that I would live. Their care for me rapidly helped me gain weight and survive the first precarious few months of life. They saw me through childhood illnesses and my day-to-day struggle to thrive. Today, in many countries, being born premature is no longer as much of a detriment as it was in the past. A premature newborn can survive and be healthy and happy as a normal baby. Babies still survive, thrive, and learn to be self-sufficient in cases where prematurity results in disabilities. I survived because of my family's care and determination.

Determination, perseverance, strength, courage in the face of adversity, and a strong will to survive are the character traits and skills that were ingrained in me as a child, and they are the foundation for the bond between my family and me that has lasted all of my life. This early training taught me life lessons about what a person can accomplish when she sets her mind to something. My family members lived by faith. My grandmother, especially, was a devout Christian. She insisted that her grandchildren would walk in the faith. She would say, "When all else is gone and you are lost, God will find you."

My family tells me that as a child, I did not like staying outdoors for long. Growing up on a tropical island, this poses a problem. Where do you go to get out of the sun? I squinted a lot and was thoroughly uncomfortable in the sun for long periods. As I grew older, I preferred activities in the house as much as possible, so I got the nickname "little mother." In a culture that celebrates women and motherhood, this was acceptable to me.

From what I know today, I was bothered by the glare. It seems that eye concerns and eye problems have dominated the female psyche in my family. We are all concerned with protecting our children's eyes. We live in fear that our children, especially our girls, will die blind, as so many women before us have done. I often wonder if, along with the blindness gene the women in my family have inherited, we have also handed down the fear gene. On exceptionally bright, sunny days, when my children were young, I always asked if they were wearing their sunglasses.

My early school years were spent in a Catholic school; one of my most vivid recollections is of one Ash Wednesday when all the children were rounded up to go to the chapel for mass. We had to cross the court-yard of our school to go to the chapel. It was a very bright and sunny day. The nuns had promised us that if we were good children, we would have a long recess that day. I remember the dread I felt at having to walk across that courtyard in all that light to reach the chapel.

I kept stumbling and falling into other children and being scolded by the nuns. When we got into the cool, dark chapel, I felt relief. I remember looking at a stained glass depiction of an angel hovering over a child as she walked on a lonely road alone. The angel was blond and blue eyed, just as the child was. The sunlight streamed through the glass in an array of beautiful colors. Yet, that day, I felt that the picture was there just for me. I hoped that an angel would be watching over me.

For all the years that I attended that school, that stained glass picture in that cool and darkened chapel was my consolation. Today, I no longer see colors, but I remember that glass window very well. Of course, I never did enjoy long recesses while at the school. I was kept indoors to do chores for being such a bumbling, stumbling student.

During my childhood in the Dominican Republic, my family lacked access to routine, affordable preventative health care. Had I been taken to an eye specialist early, some visual testing may have provided some answers to my extreme sensitivity to light. Although the science and research into eye conditions was in developing stages, my case may have garnered some interest among eye specialists. In my family, as with the majority of other Dominican families, most of our illnesses were cured at home. My grandmother and aunt had a home remedy for whatever ailed us, which generally worked.

It was not until I was brought to the United States as a preteen that I had regular contact with health care providers. I had my first dental and eye checkups at that time, and I had already been experiencing dental and eye problems. We lived in a low-income housing community commonly referred to as the projects. Life in the projects was not easy for anyone, especially when an immigrant teen. Most of us who grew up in the projects only survived, thrived, and were successful through the sheer force of will and determination. In addition, we had the help of teachers and counselors in the schools, church, and community organizations and social programs.

One of the important things to understand about poverty is that a person who does not have access to health care does not understand basic health care procedures. Things as simple as how to take proper care of the body are not a priority for someone who is struggling just to survive. So, for the first time in my life, I was sent to the dentist. I was not aware of dental procedures. Despite our language differences, the dentist helped me understand that I needed to have my teeth filled. Even after he showed me the implements to be used, namely a drill, I did not fully understand the implications.

My mother, like many immigrants to the United States, worked several jobs to make ends meet. Money for dentists and eye specialists was important, but not as high a priority as keeping a roof over our heads and food on the table. She placed high value on education and work. Unless it was absolutely necessary to go to the doctor, we generally maintained our health the best way we could. For many immigrants in the United States, gaining access to health insurance or health programs was as difficult then as it is today. Schools, churches, and community action programs helped families such as ours with health care services. We were lucky to have help from church members and friends in our community.

The first time an eye specialist saw me, I was diagnosed with astigmatism and was told I needed glasses. I am inclined to believe that this diagnosis was partially correct, given the fact that I was eventually diagnosed with Cone Rod Dystrophy. The research on retinal dysfunctions was not as advanced as it is today. In addition, I did not have the appropriate language to articulate my symptoms adequately. It seems clear to me now that there should have been much more conversation and testing done regarding my symptoms.

Parents who have children with eye issues must research their children's symptoms. Being observant and keeping track of the child's complaints, relative to what the child can actually see or not see, is also very important. Relaying this information to the eye doctor instigates an interest to examine the situation further. For me, as a preteen, the only part of that conversation was, "she needs glasses," along with, "she needs braces," which no teenager, regardless of where he/she comes from, wants to hear. These were fatal words o a young person then, but needing glasses and braces is much more common and acceptable now. Back then, it was especially noxious for an immigrant child trying to fit in. Throughout the years that I lived in New Jersey, I continued experiencing extreme light sensitivity and an aversion to light of any kind. Photos taken over those years show definite squinting, especially of my left eye. I was routinely having eye checkups and being told that I had twenty-twenty vision. As a fully sighted person, I was able to continue my high school education, work, graduate from high school, and attend university. It was not until that fateful day when I noticed floaters and dark spots in my eyes that I thought I had something more to worry about.

CHAPTER 2:
THE TELLTALE EFFECTS
OF A RETINAL PROBLEM

Spots, specks, floaters, flecks, and flashes, too

I waited in glorious anticipation for the start of the new school year. I enjoyed the days of calm before the energy that would come with the first day of school. During these quiet days, teachers typically received course and room assignments, student rolls, other assigned duties, and materials for the coming year. There was the camaraderie of the school wide general meeting, which officially began the school year. Teachers would attend this meeting en masse. It was mandatory, but it gave us the opportunity to catch up with friends and meet new teachers. Back in our schools, there were general staff meetings, department meetings, and finally individual content meetings to attend. All of these had the goal of informing and preparing teachers for the differing local, state, and federal mandates, and assigned duties, responsibilities, and new targets and goals for the teachers and students. After all the seemingly endless activities, it was time for the teacher to be alone with his/her thoughts and be free to organize and to exercise their creativity and perfect their craft. Teachers could begin the business of preparing classrooms with serious, joyful intent and renewed energy, and most importantly, we could prepare and fortify ourselves physically and emotionally for the first bell of the first day of the school year.

It always felt like a grand homecoming to start the school year. Once the classes began, I enjoyed the challenge of learning all I could about my students: their learning styles, family history, strengths, and challenges. I especially liked the creativity involved in planning and implementing lesson plans and just getting into the rhythm of school. Schools have a "flow" of their own that is palpable. Schools have an individuality that can be felt as soon as one walks through the front doors. A visitor can quickly discern whether a school is welcoming, nurturing, and effective, or whether the opposite is true. This vibe is obvious in the way one is greeted by staff members at the front office, in the hallways, or just the general appearance of the school itself. Little things such as posters and signs on the school walls give a lot of information about what the school is like. The lack of welcoming signs or evidence of multilingual signs directing visitors create an ambience, whether intended or not by the school.

In 1993, I approached the beginning of the school year with exuberance, just as I always did. I relished the fact that my life was following the plan I had set for myself. It was my pride and joy to be secure in the knowledge that I had found my niche after all. I was proud of being a classroom teacher.

This was also an important year because although my professional life was rising to new heights, my marriage of almost twenty years was ending. Despite the sadness of this loss that our family went through and subsequent emotional turmoil for my children and me, we were able to meet the challenges inherent in a divorce. My children and I gradually worked through our feelings of sadness and loss together. We settled into new routines and a new reality. My children were doing well in school and were active in sports and other school activities. To my amazement and heartfelt gratitude, they strove to be understanding of the situation and were supportive of each other and of me. As many single parents do, I spent my days working, and after work, devoting myself to the needs of my children.

There were after-school activities to drive them to, homework to complete, dinner to prepare, and nighttime rituals of assurances to get through. After they had gone to sleep, there were papers to grade and lesson plans to write for the next day of classes. The days, weeks, and years, flew by in a flurry of driving around our county from one activity to the next. On any given day, I would be up by five in the morning and fall into bed around midnight. It was the typical life of a single mother. Curiously, there was a kind of comfort in knowing that I could make life work for us on my own. The moments at dawn and late at night felt as though time was suspended—as if I had been caught in a sort of bubble where everything slowed down and I could catch my breath. I could also keenly experience my aloneness during these times. Solitude is sometimes welcome; feeling alone, I think, never is.

I spent these early morning hours in the kitchen putting together lunches, drinking the first cup of coffee of the day, and running my lesson plans in my mind. I called it the calming time. I could take this time to plan things out. During these peaceful mornings in 1993, after my divorce, I felt time stretching out before me like a clean white sheet. It reminded me of the days we would wash bed sheets in the Dominican Republic. My grandmother would set up two washbasins—one for washing and the other for rinsing. After working for hours up to our elbows in soapsuds and bluing rinse water in the unrelenting heat of the day, we hung the white sheets on clothes lines in the patio or the backyard. They would quickly dry under the hot sun. It was satisfying to see the results—no stains or wrinkles.

This is how I pictured my life during that year, like pure white sheets in my mind, just waiting for whatever new images my life would bring. My future, and that of my children, was mine to design. I began to keep a journal. I wanted to write down as much as I could about how I felt and what was happening to my family during this and the coming transformative years. As it turned out, this journal became an important tool for my eye specialist. As I recorded the changes I was experiencing in my life, I also included those changes that were occurring to my vision. These entries helped my eye specialist gather valuable information that aided her in screening and diagnosing my condition.

It was during this time that I decided to go back to graduate school and finish a master's degree that I had begun working toward in 1981. My son was born that year, and my priorities shifted. But in 1993, trying to put my divorce behind me, going back to school offered me what I felt was a fresh start. I found meaning and purpose in my life again. Attending graduate school also provided, in retrospect, a reason for why I did not pay as much attention as I should have to my changing vision. Even as I focused on restoring my life, I was gradually losing my eyesight. The irony of this is that I was losing my vision while gaining insight and clarity about what I was doing and how I wanted to prepare a future for my children and me. I suppose that I was so busy planning for life that I missed, or perhaps ignored, the changes and therefore the opportunity to do what I could early on to know and learn about my eye disorder.

From time to time, though, I would see, or rather perceive, annoying things like squiggly lines floating in my eyes. There were spots, specks, and streamers. There were floaters, flashes, and flecks. But since my yearly vision exams were always great, I was told time and again that my vision was twenty-twenty, so it was easy to ignore these things drifting aimlessly around in my field of vision. However, I routinely discussed them with the optometrist that I saw regularly, but I was told that ordinary eye floaters and spots are very common and usually did not warrant cause for alarm.

In retrospect, the optometrist should have referred me right away to a specialist in retinal problems. I would have learned what I have since learned on my own. As I researched what is known about flashes and floaters in the eyes, I learned that most people experience spots and floaters. These are usually confined to a particular part of the eye and can be made to disappear with eye movements. Floaters and spots can often appear when very small pieces of the eye's vitreous matter break loose within the inner back portion of the eye. Spots and floaters may not necessarily indicate that there is an eye disorder; however, a consultation with an eye specialist is recommended.

Flashes in the eye look like bright points that appear with the eyes open or closed. These points of light will "flash" in a circular fashion around the center of the eye. These flashes will appear in one eye and last for an instant. When flashes are present in the eye, this can be a sign of some kind of eye disorder. A specialist should be seen immediately.

When we are young, the vitreous matter has a gel-like consistency. However, as we age, the vitreous matter dissolves and liquefies. It loses its viscosity to create a watery center. Some of this matter occasionally will float around in the more liquid center of the vitreous matter as a result of this process. These pieces look like floating web-like strings.

During one of those calm, early morning times, I realized that there was something odd going on in my left eye. I reflected on this briefly but quickly ignored it as the hustle and bustle of the new day began. That faithful morning, everything went on as usual. I was up early, made lunches for my children, and got them off to school. It was a bright, sunny, fall day, and I was enjoying the drive to work. When I was not busy running through my lesson plans in my head, I took note of the bright fall colors, which adorned the world and filled my field of vision. In later years, I have often been thankful that I had taken the time to notice the beauty of nature. These are now memories to me since I will never again see the colors of a day in fall, blue skies, or the blue-green of the Caribbean Sea.

But on this day, I quite suddenly sensed a change in my vision. The world seemed momentarily "off" somehow. I closed one eye and then the other, and that is when I noticed that in my left eye, these spots and floaters were particularly pronounced. Against the background of the bright, clear sky, I could see them plainly, and most alarmingly, my left eye seemed dimmer to me than my right eye.

I immediately made an appointment to see the optometrist, and this time he suggested I see an ophthalmologist. What I have come to know is that you can't actually see tiny bits of broken off gel-like pieces of vitreous floating loose within your eye. What you see instead, are the shadows from these floaters as they appear on the retina. As your eyes move, these floaters also move around creating the illusion that they are drifting around aimlessly in your eyes. The truly amazing thing is that we become accustomed to having these conditions and telling ourselves that they are nothing serious. We simply hope that they go away. For a very long time, and since I had twenty-twenty vision, as I had been told, I did nothing about it.

I finally saw the ophthalmologist in 1996, and so began a journey of discovery that lasted five years before I could receive a diagnosis. By 1996, I was seeing floaters and spots regularly, which were sometimes accompanied by light flashes.

Many years after my diagnosis, I was referred by one of my ophthalmologists to the National Institutes of Health for field of vision screenings. I remember one doctor at the NIH telling me that the flashes were the attempts by my retina to adjust to light coming into my eyes. The truth is much more alarming. The appearance of these flashes could mean that the vitreous is pulling away from the retina. It could very well mean that the retina itself is becoming detached from the inner back of the eye. A detached retina or any number of other problems related to the interference with the healthy functioning of the retina is a serious emergency. In cases of retinal tear or detachment, eye infections or eye surgery, medical action must be taken as soon as possible so that an eye surgeon can reattach the retina and restore eye function before vision is lost permanently.

One of the most important factors in this process of determining what is wrong with your eyes is the access to good healthcare that an individual has. If an individual does not have access to good vision care, the chances are that such treatable eye conditions, when left unattended, will lead to more complications, and perhaps even adverse and negative outcomes. There are credited reports that state that perhaps three hundred million people worldwide are blind or visually impaired simply because they don't have access to good eye care.

I was fortunate in that I had health insurance, which included access to excellent vision care. I was able to see eye specialist at some of the most important and prestigious centers in my area as well as in the United States. My ophthalmologist was at the Georgetown Center for Sight. She referred me to John Hopkins for additional testing and second opinions. I also saw doctors at George Washington University, The Retina Group, and The National Institute of Health Eye Clinic. It is evident that because I was a teacher with good health insurance, I was seen by some of the best doctors in order to take care of my eye problems. I also had one of the rarest conditions in the area of retinal conditions, which no doubt raised quite a bit of intellectual curiosity and interest on the part of these doctors.

Thus, the road to determining what was wrong with my eyes began with a conversation with the Georgetown Center for Sight ophthalmologist. The very first request was for a detailed description of what I had been experiencing. Fortunately, I had been keeping detailed notes in my journal regarding all that was happening to my eyes. The conversation that we had gave me the opportunity to share all the personal reporting that I had documented. This in turn gave her the chance to theorize about what we might find, and most importantly, where to begin the process of discovery, and what tests to order. Next, the doctor turned her attention to the records that she had asked to be transferred to her from my optometrist. These records were instrumental in demonstrating the status of my eye examinations over time, which established a baseline for the doctor to follow. Once again, the fact that I had been able to have regular eye exams every year for a number of years helped to move the process along. The records from the optometrist were also as helpful as my own personal records.

Having health insurance assured a continuity of care that is essential. It may be inconvenient to gather and keep medical records or have these transferred from one doctor to another, but these are necessary activities. The professional's data and screenings are the support to the individual's firsthand accounting of the problem. Together, the science and the personal insight move the process along more quickly. I probably shortened the years it would have taken to receive my diagnosis. Five years is a long time to wait for an answer, but as I learned, it is usual when faced with an unknown condition.

In many cases, the illness or condition may already have a battery of tests and a field of knowledge, which aid in the resulting diagnosis. Finding the underlying cause of an individual's condition will take much longer when there is not a lot of research in the field, and/or the condition is rare. However, research and technologies are constantly improving in many fields, including that of challenging eye conditions. As larger groups of individuals with hard to diagnose conditions are identified, more research protocols and studies are done. There is hope that these studies will shed light on the kind of treatments that may be available to patients in the near future.

In the meantime, patients must be proactive and engaged in the discovery process and in learning about whatever treatment methods are available. Being proactive and engaged initially means paying attention to the changes in your body, keeping personal records of what you are experiencing, having conversations with your doctor, and doing research on your own—in short, becoming enlightened. Having an illness or condition alter the course of your life is overwhelming and traumatic. Actually taking charge and being engaged in this process of discovery is not only enlightening, but it also is empowering. Being enlightened and feeling empowered has been extremely helpful to me as I physically adjusted to blindness. As I worked along with my doctors, and we found solutions to problems I encountered in my daily tasks, I felt strong emotionally as well. The doctors were working on my behalf, and I was, too.

The visual field tests that were given to me revealed a number of problem areas. There were dark spots in my eyes, which I learned were called scotomas. They were found off to the side of my eyes in the periphery fields. New spots were discovered as we progressed through the various visual field tests. Early tests proved that there was one scotoma in my left eye, but soon more were found. As we progressed through the detective-like work of trying to find out what type of eye problem I had, other spots appeared. It was clear to me that my left eye would be completely overtaken by these spots. In addition, I had poor central acuity, which continued to progress. With the advent of time, the ability of my eyes to perceive color also diminished.

Although overwhelming in the implications of what I was learning, clearly I was going blind, I was still much amazed by the imagery presented in the graphs that these visual fields produced. I had dreams where these scotoma looked somewhat like what I envisioned were the depictions of black holes in space. In my dreams, the dark spots in my eyes acted as a vacuum that slowly absorbed the healthy spaces of my eyes, my body, and my mind, leaving behind a total void. In panic, I would wake up thinking that this was the day that I would be totally blind. But each day I woke with the reality of a progressive and gradual deterioration of my sight, rather than sudden and total blindness. Clearly, I had to work on driving myself into sheer panic. I truly appreciated the reasoned voice of my ophthalmologist in these moments. She would calm my fears and review the data with me. She explained the phenomena that were occurring and the possible reasons for them. I asked questions and developed strategies to cope with the challenges I was beginning to experience. Quite quickly, the first challenge presented was how to deal with the extreme photophobia—sensitivity to light—that was causing real hardship for me in the classroom. This has been the most uncomfortable effect of Cone Rod Dystrophy to manage.

The question of how much central acuity I was losing was the next area of concern. I began to notice that when grading my student's homework, and in other tasks where I had to read documents, I was experiencing a lot of disturbance. One day, rather than seeing words on a page, I saw what looked like little ants marching across the page. I looked up from what I was doing in panic and looked all around me. Everything else in the world looked normal to me. The student's desks, my desks, the closet, and the classroom windows—everything was the same—but I knew that was the last day that I would be able to work on my student's papers without assistive technology.

We began a series of tests that the eye specialist felt were necessary to do in order to discover what was happening with my eyes. I have found that it was helpful to know a little about the tests that are to be done so that one can be actively engaged in the decision making process. An MRI, EKG, ERG, along with neurological and blood tests, are most commonly prescribed by eye specialists. Getting to know what each of these tests is designed to do is very important. Ii is just as crucial to inquire about what is to be done. Never be afraid to ask questions of the doctor when you don't understand something. I have found in some cases that the way in which the doctor has answered my questions has helped me determine if I want that individual as my doctor.

MRI stands for Magnetic Resonance Imaging. This a tool used for diagnostic purposes. An MRI machine is used to scan the part of the body to be diagnosed. The diagnostic machine utilizes magnetic fields and radio waves to attract the water in the portion of the body under study in order to create images.

This kind of tool is very good at detecting issues that are occurring in soft body tissues. It is often used to find tumors and other such conditions in areas such as the brain, spinal cord, heart, and eyes. The ophthalmologist will determine whether you require an MRI and what to expect when you go for the appointment.

EKG refers to an electrocardiogram. This test checks the functioning of the heart. The heart emits electrical pulses when it beats, and these electrical impulses can be recorded on the EKG machine. The actual purpose is to determine whether the heart is beating with a normal rhythm or if there are underlying heart problems. Clearly, this kind of test is best used to discover any heart problems, but in the case of eye conditions, it can also be useful to determine if blood pressure is involved in the eye problem. It may be that high blood pressure/hypertension is affecting how the eyes are functioning. Another indicator is whether there are mineral deficiencies in the blood. The eye specialist will review and interpret what the EKG record is demonstrating.

An ERG or electroretinography is an eye test that is used to determine how the retina is functioning. The retina is the part of the eye that detects light. This test is designed to examine the functioning of the cones and rods. The test consists of placing something akin to a contact lens on the cornea, which is located in the front of the eye. Electrodes are placed in precise positions on the skin in order to measure the responses of the cones and rods to light stimulus. These very light electrical impulses are recorded and interpreted by the eye specialist. This tool helps the eye specialist find what type of retinal condition the patient has. It can further verify whether the condition is inherited or acquired. Very often, this type of test will indicate if surgery is needed. An example would be the presence of cataracts.

Utilizing the data from these varied tests, my eye specialist was able to systematically rule out many eye disorders, such as those relating to the optic nerves. Optic neuritis is a well-known example of one of these disorders. The tests were able to point accurately to the problem residing within the retina. The ah-ha moment was achieved when the eye specialist used a retinal-imaging camera to take pictures of the back of the eye. These new instruments, often called an Optomap or Retinal Imaging System, have the capacity to show a panoramic view of the entire inner eye. These pictures can be taken without the need for dilation, which makes this a more comfortable experience for the patient. With this added to all of the tests at the disposal of the eye specialist, the chances of arriving at a diagnosis are greatly improved.

This is not to say that there won't be a misdiagnosis. I have learned that many eye problems have similar symptoms. They are so similar that only the skill of the ophthalmologist and the appropriate testing mechanisms can ferret out the truth. I was privileged to have a doctor that had done extensive work with retinal disorders and had many years of experience with different types of retinal conditions. In fact, my eye specialist had published works in the area of cone and rod dysfunction. It is a godsend to find a competent doctor who is also confident enough in his or her skills to refer you to other doctors for second and third opinions.

Initial attempts at a diagnosis were made after a few tests were run. Optic neuritis and retinopathy were ruled out, as were common diseases, such as cataracts and glaucoma. Tests were done for the possibility of HIV/AIDS, diabetes, hypertension, multiple sclerosis, and even Lyme disease. After years of testing and exploring one avenue and another, my ophthalmologist was finally able to determine that I had Cone Rod Dystrophy. The euphoria that I felt at that moment, to finally learn what was wrong, was dashed moments later when she informed me that unfortunately, there was no cure for the condition. Like most people in the world, I believed that diagnosis would lead to treatment and relief. It is a rude awakening to find out that many of the ills that we suffer are not fixable. In fact, many conditions, such as Cone Rod Dystrophy, are still vastly unknown to medical professionals. To date, it is not known how Cone Rod Dystrophy develops in families. It is unknown which genes are involved in the presentation of this condition.

Cone Rod Dystrophy is said to be a genetic/inherited disorder, or it can be an acquired condition. It can be stable or progressive in nature, leading to severe visual impairment, substantial loss of vision, and blindness. What no doctor can or won't say is whether it will also lead to total blindness. The point, however, is immaterial to the patient living with Cone Rod Dystrophy. Whether stable or progressive, the loss of vision is summarily life altering. The individual must learn coping strategies to deal with blindness in its essence. Strategies for coping physically, mentally, socially, and emotionally will be important to acquire.

One of the important and early ways to cope is to retrace one's family medical history. I found this a worthwhile activity on many levels. It helped to systematically eliminate certain medical possibilities. For example, glaucoma, diabetes, and cataracts were present in many of my family members. Incidents of cancer, multiple sclerosis, and lupus were rare or not present at all. High blood pressure/hypertension, anemia, and other blood related conditions were also present among some people in my family. A major reason, then, for the passage of so much time in determining the   diagnosis had to do with eliminating potential issues and concentrating on what conditions were possible for me to inherit.

The tests were important, but costly and time consuming. Patients who have a clear understanding of their family medical history, who keep track of their experiences with the condition, have health insurance or access to health programs, and who receive regular eye care will succeed in gaining a diagnosis and the likely prognosis. The hope is that this process will lead to what treatments/cures are available, or at the very least, what options are present.

Receiving the diagnosis and possible prognosis for the future is not the end of the journey; it's only the beginning. It was devastating to learn that there was no way to cure my eyes. Our society clings to the hope that everything that ails us can be fixed. Therefore, it is traumatic to learn that one of my most precious senses was going to continue to deteriorate. No clock can tell you how, when, or where you will simply stop seeing everything that is dear to you. The faces of your loved ones, your surroundings, the colors of life, and even your hearing, will all start to fade over time. The questioning period begins.

For months after my diagnosis, I questioned and debated with myself endlessly. What had I done to deserve this fate? Had I done this to myself somehow? How would I move on with life? What quality of life would I have? What would be my limitations? Who are the people available to help and support me? How would I continue to be independent? How was I going to break the news to my loved ones? These thoughts went on and on in endless variations. At forty-five years of age, I was faced with having to map out a new blueprint for what I would do next in my life. It seemed a daunting task. I also understood that I needed the help of the doctors in the field to build a new framework for living with my visual impairment.

There were times during this period when I indulged in circular thinking, which lead to negativity and anxiety. Too many times, I played the "what if" game in my mind: What if I had early access to health care and had been taken to an eye specialist as a child? What if I had been born in the United States with better opportunities for good health care and nutrition? Was my prematurity a factor in my disability? Could my family's socioeconomic status and the fact that I grew up in poverty have exacerbated the condition? Or, did growing up an Upward Bound project kid in New Jersey limit my opportunities for receiving better health care? In retrospect, I lost valuable time in this negative and irrational mode of thought. I could have spent the same time informing myself about how to manage the eye disorder in ways that lead to more positive thinking and joyful living.

The strongest argument that can be made for providing people with access to good health insurance is that good health care provides rational, healthy mental states. Knowing what the illness is, how it affects the individual, and what options and solutions are available go a long way in creating a more positive outlook. It is evident that early detection and diagnosis of most illnesses will lead to a better understanding of what options are available for treating patients. It follows that those who have access to the possibility of better care will have more treatment options. The potential for providing positive outcomes and survival for such patients is greatly improved. For adults experiencing life altering illnesses and conditions, positive outcomes mean longevity and high productivity. Although, in the case of genetic conditions, such as Cone Rod Dystrophy, there are no cures, there is the promise of continued effectiveness as a productive member of the workforce and of society. That is cause for optimism and hope for the future. In the end, all humans expect to be able to pursue a life that is full of hope and joy.

My experiences as a parent, teacher, and social services worker have afforded me keen affinity to the plight of families with children. Parents who have children affected by severe illnesses and challenging conditions are among the most vulnerable of populations. Early access to preventative health care and opportunities for adequate treatments cannot be understated. In particular, parents with children who have Cone Rod Dystrophy need to initiate an early intervention. The earlier the intervention and diagnosis, the earlier appropriate treatment can be applied. Parents are able to provide a healthier lifestyle for their children when they are equipped with knowledge of the condition and have access to the available methods for treatment.

It is important to determine the nature of the condition or illness so that other family members, who may also be affected in the future, can be forewarned and forearmed. In addition, the patient, when faced with overwhelming and life-altering information, may need to draw emotional support from family members. Health professionals who are engaged in the care of the individual are great stores of information and support, and are knowledgeable about necessary resources. Seeking the aid of support groups and others in the community who show interest in educating and employing individuals with conditions such as a visual impairment are resources that the affected individual and her family will need. Therefore, to begin the process of understanding what the ailment is, what options are available, and what management of the illness or condition entails, adults and children need to tap into the knowledge that these professionals have.

In the life of an individual with visual impairment, many people will have questions about what is happening to the person they know and love. Parents with school-age children in particular are also faced with adults in the school who want to have some clear understanding as to how to assist the child. To help a child cope with his visual issues and to allow him to feel comfortable around other children is a testament to how well the parents and the school staff are communicating. The fact is that all of these individuals in our lives need to be aware of the causes, symptoms, and effects that our visual impairments have on us.

A famous cliché states that knowledge is power. I often think that knowledge gives you the power to discuss your condition with authority. Being one's own advocate means that one has to be knowledgeable enough to inform others effectively. Self-advocacy is empowering. This helps the individuals affected in meaningful ways because they will be able to discuss the illness or condition in a more natural and informed way. This ability will set the listener at ease. The affected individual feels more confident and competent, and therefore, more able to inform others of the strategies, tools, and assistance he will need without feeling that he is a burden. Finally, the affected individual can anticipate and better cope with the inevitable debilitating effects of the condition. This confidence will translate into the power to address the people in the individual's life with the needs that arise, the limitations that may become present, and the necessary accommodations that need to be made when the time finally comes. Teachers, family members, health professionals, and employers, to name a few, may be relieved to know that the individual has taken an active role in managing a new life as a blind person. When you have become blind-sighted, you will no longer be blindsided by the reality of losing your vision.

To understand what it is to become blind by Cone Rod Dystrophy, we must know what being sighted means. Simply, we see what our brains wants us to see, or rather the signals our eyes see in the external world go to our brain to be "translated" into things that make sense. Our brain is the sight center. Poets and thinkers have said that our eyes are a window to the soul. Practically speaking, our eyes are a window for our brains. In essence, the eyes relay images as light impulses gathered through parts of the eyes. Each part has a distinct role to play in putting together the information that will travel to the brain for translation. Light is the way in which images are conducted through the front of the eyes to the back of the eye.

To understand what is taking place in Cone Rod Dystrophy, or any eye disorder for that matter, it is necessary to be knowledgeable of the anatomy of the eye. I confess that I had nothing but a rudimentary knowledge of the parts of the eye. I quickly had to take a crash course in what each part was and what it was designed to do. To understand what Cone Rod Dystrophy is, one must know what the eyes are designed to do. The eye has three basic components: the front of the eye, the back of the eye, and the optic nerve. Each component has individual parts that provide a necessary function to the productivity of the eye. The front of the eye contains the cornea, the lens, the pupil, and the iris. These structures focus the light entering the eye and direct it to the second component of the eye, the retina, which is a light sensitive area located at the back of the eye that acts much like the film of a camera. It is interesting to note that Retina was also the name given to a photographic camera designed and built by the Germans. It was widely popular during and after World War II. Its popularity was due to its compact size and the use of the then new 35 mm film. The brand name was Kodak, which continues to be a popular brand today. The name given to this camera may have been in tribute to the perfect design of the retina in the eye. This film in our eyes not only manages the light that is reflected there, but also provides the clarity, contrast, and color that humans need in order to see well.

The final component can be thought of as the conductor of the light that has gone through the retina and been translated for use by the brain. This structure is known as the optic nerve. It acts as a wire that conducts the coded light from the retina to the brain. A person is able to see fully when these components work together. Occasionally, some part of the eye will not be functioning properly due to a genetic flaw or an acquired condition. Conditions that cause challenges to a person's vision can be found in the front of the eye or from problems with the optic nerve. Most common are ailments such as myopia, astigmatism, conjunctivitis, achromatopsia, cataracts, glaucoma, retinopathy, and optic neuritis.

Knowledge of the anatomy of the eye does not stop with the general components. One should also know something regarding the inner workings of the parts of the eye. Light comes through the lens of the eye and is focused by the cornea. The light then passes through a hole called the pupil. A circle of muscle referred to as the iris surrounds the pupil. The iris is the colored part of the eye. The light is then focused onto the back of the eye by a lens. Very small, light sensitive structures called photoreceptors cover the back of the eye much like film in a camera. These photoreceptors collect information about the visual world.

Rods and cones are the two types of photoreceptors. Their names stem from their forms, which can be viewed through a microscope. Rods enable people to see things that move. Because we have rods in our eyes, we perceive the movement of a car or the hands on a clock. We are also able to see in the dark. When rods are functioning at their capacity, we can even distinguish very dark items from not so dark ones against the background of the night. However, rods do not have the capacity to let us see at night in color. We can only see items in black and white and in less detail.

The cones in our eyes allow us to see things that are standing still. We are able to see in daylight since one of the main functions of the cones is to filter light. Cones allow us to see in color and in fine detail. The millions of rod and cone photoreceptors at the back of the eye make up the thin film that is the retina. In the case of Cone Rod Dystrophy, the patient gradually loses acuity in the center of the vision field. The reason for this is that the central portion of the retina is made up solely of cones. They help us see the central bit of vision that we use for reading, looking at photographs and recognizing faces. The area of the retina around the central bit is made up of rods. The rods see the surrounding bits of vision and help us to walk around and not bump into things, especially in the dark. The signals that cones and rods decipher are sent to the brain through the wires that make up each optic nerve. The optic nerves are literally wired to the brain. To be sighted then means that all parts of the brain and eye are working at full capacity for us to see normally.

Most people tend to take health for granted. If it does not hurt, all must be well. The proliferation of health maintenance programs provided through health insurance carriers has forced most of us to consider the error in our judgment. Annual check-ups and routine examinations and screenings are more of the norm today. We take our senses even more for granted than perhaps other parts of our bodies. We expect them to work with little or no special care. We get our annual vision exam, and we're good to go. During our annual physical, our ears, noses, and throats are checked very quickly. Do we even have a check up for our sense of taste and touch? Somehow, seeing, smelling, tasting, touching, and hearing don't seem to be that big of a deal—until they are lost. As long as they are doing what they are intended to do, or they are not affected by some illness, we don't pay much attention.

I have come to realize that the old adage, "You don't know what you have until it's gone," is oh so true. It saves time, money, and worry to visit the doctor and be assured that everything is in working order. Particularly in the case of retinal conditions, it pays to have an examination of the front and back of the eyes.

Cone Rod Dystrophy is a name given to a wide range of eye conditions that involve the retina. These eye conditions are all linked by a problem with the cone and rod photoreceptors found in this area of the eye. Although the term dystrophy is used for conditions that are present at birth, the photoreceptors, in this case, either do not work from birth, or else slowly stop working over time. In addition, there are studies available that report startling evidence of degeneration in other areas due to the eye problem. The condition may affect other parts of the body. One's hearing may also degenerate over time because of an eye disorder.

The cause of the degeneration of the cone and rod photoreceptors is not always clear. There can be many genetic implications as well as the nature of the disorder's onset. Every case is different and particular to an individual's physiology. Extensive screening and testing is the first step is diagnosis. Most reported cases, however, are caused by defects in the genes that control the cones and rods. Genes are thought of as chemical markers or blueprints, which we have stored in our body. These markers direct and tell all of our body parts how to work correctly. Another way to look at genes is as the body's system of maps. If a gene has a misprint or defect in its blueprint, then a part of the body may not work properly. Individuals with Cone Rod Dystrophy inherit or acquire this malfunctioning gene from one or both parents, or by some quirk in the individual's physical development.

In other words, this malfunction of a gene may be a consequence of the person's own body. Thus, some people do not inherit the gene defect, but for unexplained reasons, they are simply born that way. The parent's genes are normal; yet, by a stroke of fate, a new "mistake" occurs in the person's genes. The new mistake is then carried to a new generation. This new defect may be passed on to the offspring of the affected individual. Currently, not all is known about how the genes malfunction or even what kind of transmittal problems there are. Much more research is needed, especially in the area of who may be in danger of inheriting or acquiring the malfunctioning gene. As an affected individual, one can only marvel at the incredible nature of human development. Because of a mistake in genetics, a malfunctioning gene gradually extinguishes the cones and rods in the eyes like so many sputtering, dying light bulbs.

In order to find out whether one has inherited a malfunctioning gene or acquired it by chance, rigorous research and genome investigation is required. I was referred to the National Institute of Health to be a part of a research study concerning this condition. The ultimate goal of the study was to determine what genes might be involved in the presentation of Cone Rod Dystrophy. The importance of this kind of study is manifold.

The research and subsequent studies may eventually lead to the identification of the malfunctioning gene. Likewise, this activity may lead scientists to develop treatments helpful in alleviating the symptoms of these conditions, or even find a cure. Since there have already been many types of Cone Rod Dystrophies identified, the challenge is to isolate the particular genes that are causing the particular effects. Among the most well-known types of Cone Rod Dystrophies are Leber's congenital amaurosis, retinitis pigmentosa, Usher's Syndrome, and Batten's disease.

Receiving a diagnosis of Cone Rod Dystrophy takes quite some time. Patients learn very early in the process that they need to be patient. In this case, patience is not only a virtue; it's a virtual necessity. An ophthalmologist must determine that the problem is in the retina and not elsewhere in the eye. Visual field tests and other screenings must be done to focus on the back of the eye and the retina.

The birth of a child is a miracle in itself. Millions of babies around the world are born every day and develop in predictable patterns. Most babies are born with no major complications or discernible differences. With the help of health care providers, a child develops normally. Parents and doctors will have a greater chance of picking up any abnormalities if the child is monitored during and after pregnancy. Access and affordability of health care, therefore, is the first line of defense in the path towards a correct diagnosis of a problem.

In young children with Cone Rod Dystrophy, the parent or the pediatrician may notice certain visual behaviors that fall outside of the norm. Among the things that may capture attention are fast to-and-fro movements of the eyes. This condition is called Nystagmus. In another condition, the eyes appear to wander around, unable to fixate on any one object. People may notice the child squinting at bright lights or touching her eyes frequently with her fingers. These kinds of abnormalities should alert parents and caregivers of the need for further investigation. Parents armed with a little knowledge may notice that their child's vision may be reduced and bring this to the doctor's attention.

When these symptoms are present, it is clearly the time for a doctor's assessment. Although some conditions turn out to be benign in nature or easily corrected, others may interfere with the child's overall development. In the case of retinal disorders, and specifically Cone Rod Dystrophy, an eye specialist can check the way the eyes behave to bright lights. If the pupils in the child's eye move slowly to a bright light, then Cone Rod Dystrophy is more likely. Using a special instrument, the eye doctor can look at the optic nerve and retina at the back of the eye. In children with this condition, sometimes these parts of the eye look different from normal eyes.

As I have learned, the optic nerve may look translucent, opaque, or milky. Doctors used these words as they examined my optic nerves. Taken in isolation, these observations may be incomplete and lead to a misdiagnosis. The work of the eye specialist may take a long time, but in the end, the chances of receiving the right diagnosis are much higher. Special testing is the most important work to be done, as previously mentioned. These tests will help determine what is wrong. As we know, these tests measure signals from the eyes when a child is shown a bright light. An electroretinogram or ERG machine records the electrical signals made by the eyes. The record of the signals will help the eye specialist decide what is wrong. If the signals are weak or absent, then Cone Rod Dystrophy is more likely.

When faced with the challenge of having a child who needs to take these tests, it is important for parents and doctors to properly explain to children what they will experience. Some tests may be uncomfortable or scary. In fact, some tests may not be appropriate given the child's age. For example, parents must let children know that an ERG involves sticky patches placed around the eyes. The sticky patches are attached to wires that lead to a machine. This kind of explanation and preparation will help alleviate any fears the child might have. Some Cone Rod Dystrophies may present initially with symptoms that have nothing to do with vision.

Conditions such as Batten's Disease may present with increasing difficulty handling objects, increasing clumsiness, gradual change in mood and personality, decreased attention span, slurred speech, and poor memory. It may be only later that a problem with vision is noticed. One of the commonly expressed concerns among some Cone Rod Dystrophy patients is that they had perfect or near perfect vision early in life. Whether the individual notices differences in one eye as opposed to the other, the urgency to be screened immediately is the same. As soon as these conditions become apparent, seek an assessment from an eye doctor—don't delay!

Cone Rod Dystrophies can affect different people in different ways. Yet, everyone, at first, will feel that their vision is normal. In particular, young children will not perceive anything to be wrong with their eyes. Children may not say anything about their vision for quite a while. They will assume that everyone is seeing things in the very same way that they are seeing the world. Older children and adults may eventually notice that their vision is blurred around the edges. They may further note that their vision is especially poor in bright light or in the dark. In fact, Cone Rod Dystrophy patients may only see brightness or bright lights, which become extremely uncomfortable the longer they are exposed to sources of light. I met a gentleman whose vision had been affected by some medication that he was prescribed. The medication affected his retina in such a way that he was extremely photophobic. So intense was his discomfort that he actually wished he was totally blind. The severity of this impairment to vision cannot be understated. Some measure of comfort is possible only when the individual is away from all light sources.

Some individuals will notice that their central vision is blurred. In addition, most colors will not appear as bright. Some people may only see the movement of large objects but fail to see smaller objects. Unfortunately, many people, as time goes on, will see very little. These are just some of the manifestations of the condition. These are signals that the person is having a problem with the cones and rods in his or her eyes, and there is an immediate need for testing. It is important to pay attention to these symptoms because one of the curiosities of this condition is that the person will not appear to be blind. Many patients are able to function especially well with this condition for a long time. Others have enough residual vision to manage most life tasks. I can recall a very curious day that I experienced long after I had been given my diagnosis. I was seeking accommodations at my place of employment so that I could continue working. A colleague came up to me as I was making my way down one of the halls at my school. The person greeted me and then waved her hand in front of my face. I had to tell her, "You know, I can see you doing that!"

Not all of your colleagues will be this insensitive, but it happens. Colleagues and others in your workplace may be aware that you have vision issues, but may not know what is wrong or how to approach you. They may not be able to appreciate the fact that you are legally blind just by looking at you. In fact, the terms totally blind, legally blind, and visually impaired are often confusing to people. The societal perceptions about the blind are often wrapped around myths and misinformation regarding what it really means to have loss of vision. Some may even think you are faking it to satisfy your own agenda. People with Cone Rod Dystrophy may manage very well at a great number of daily tasks, but the fact is that they do not see well.

There are quite a few differences among people with Cone Rod Dystrophy, and retinal disorders can present in a variety of ways. Visual impairment ranges from variable levels of residual vision to total blindness. Even among the visually impaired, there are variations and different symptoms. Many may also have poor hearing, learning challenges, and even stunted growth and development. Early on, I discovered that blindness was a physical condition that impacts one's entire sense of self and personal well-being. Who you perceive yourself to be influences how you feel about yourself and your surroundings. The individual who is going blind will experience existential conflicts. On the one hand, the experience is so overwhelming that almost at once, one experiences an emotional rollercoaster. Feelings of bewilderment, denial, despondency, anger, and acceptance are constant companions. Above all is a feeling of helplessness and fear derived from what we imagine will be the need to depend on others.

I went through a period where I alternated between blaming myself and fate for what was happening to my eyesight. In my mind, I convinced myself that my eyesight was instrumental in my being a success in life. I was angry because an important sense that I depended upon for determining my place in life was failing me. My ability to interact accurately with the physical environment was predicated on my ability to see well. As long as I could see and gauge everything accurately and effectively, I would be a success, and so goes the negative cyclical thinking.

The truth is that I felt my eyes were the means by which others saw me as intelligent, productive, and a valuable human being. Through my use of my eyes, I read great books, carried out my tasks as a teacher, and imparted to my students the knowledge I gained through reading. My eyes allowed me to write articles published in educational journals, by which I could share what I knew about education with others in my field. Socially, my eyes allowed me to enjoy outings to restaurants where I could easily read the menu, go to the movies to see the latest film, or just go to the supermarket to pick up groceries, but these activities had seemingly become difficult challenges. The social, psychological, and emotional conflicts, stresses, and anxieties caused by the loss of vision seem insurmountable at times.

Severe visual impairment and blindness validate that as human beings, we need to be seen as capable, intelligent, and of value to the society. The blind still need to be needed, interact with our loved ones and our environment, work, love, and enjoy life. Going blind does not mean that one goes numb. The very opposite is the case. Going blind awakens in us all of the existential reasons why we eventually must strive to carry on. What many of us struggle with is the "how" of the matter.

There is a very real conflict between the existential urge to move forward and our fear of doing so. In large measure, how we view ourselves—and indeed, how others will relate to us as blind individuals—depends on how we are able to resolve this conflict.

There is no doubt that going blind engenders among many, feelings of anxiety, stress, and fear. It certainly means adjusting to and learning to live with certain specialized conditions. Regardless of whether one is totally blind or visually impaired, one needs to learn strategies and new skills to manage life. In essence, we are presented with a new reality. Akin to having experienced the death of a loved one, loss of a limb, battles with chronic illness, or natural disasters, the journey into blindness requires an understanding of and reconciliation with the feelings that naturally occur. It becomes time to channel as much energy, enthusiasm, and effort into learning how to manage the manifestations of the condition physically, emotionally, and psychologically. The objective is to gain the knowledge and skills necessary, which will determine the level of productivity you will continue to enjoy as you journey into blindness.

The battle with feelings of loss, anxiety, despondency, and self-recrimination can be as debilitating as the condition itself. These feelings arise for many reasons. I believe, in my case, that they arose because I thought I could not continue to do all of the things that I used to do, or the things that I'd taken for granted. I felt I had to change my life goals. I wanted to be in control of every facet of my life. To me, being in control of my life meant that I was productive, and therefore, I was a valuable member of society. These feelings of inadequacy were compounded by the fact that I was entering into menopause, whose issues solidified in my mind that these changes were all bad. It just seemed as if my life was deteriorating at a fast pace.

In addition, the usual events of life were beginning to occur as well. I was faced with the issues surrounding my parents' old age. My daughter was diagnosed with cancer. A number of personal and external challenges were seemingly presenting themselves each day. At one of my low points, it seemed easy to retreat into feeling inadequate. I was going blind after all, so I would think to myself *Why bother—I can't do that anymore.* Becoming dependent on my children and others seemed like an attractive alternative. Once I started thinking along this path, these negative and irrational thoughts seemed plausible, doable, and difficult to overcome.

What I failed to recognize at that time was that I should have been taking advantage of these opportunities in order to develop as a person. There was no overwhelming difference between a sighted person and me at this stage of life. All of us must contend with change of life issues, whether man or woman. The sexes may experience aging and change of life effects differently, but we go through them nevertheless. It was simply time for me to experience personal and spiritual growth. It was also the perfect time to learn new skills and new ways to confront life's challenges.

I understood that I had been fairly stagnant in my development; I was so comfortable with my life, following the plan I had set for myself, that I never envisioned any kind of shake up. I assumed things were going to continue as usual. I was blindsided by Cone Rod Dystrophy, and this changed my way of thinking. The diagnosis and subsequent management of the condition was the catalyst for change. Not only did my way of thinking change, but I also became more prepared for the second half of my life. The more I followed this line of reasoning, the quicker those negative feelings dissipated. I became more hopeful.

There are no medicines, surgeries, or treatments yet known to correct Cone Rod Dystrophy. Although there is no stopping the loss of vision, there is good news for patients with the condition. Many strategies can be used to assist you as you lose your vision. These strategies will make it easier to see things with residual vision. You can learn to shield your eyes from bright light if your cones are not working. You learn ways to cope in the dark if your rods are the problem. You can learn to live your life on your terms simply by applying new ways to do things.

Gradually, a transformation will take place in one's thinking and behavior. Consequently, you will live a healthier, happier life with the vision you have. Life continues to be good when you are able to enjoy your family, friends, and holidays, fall in and out of love, and experience the enjoyment and the challenges of your work.

Whatever is meaningful to you can continue to be so. It just takes learning strategies and skills to navigate and articulate your experience to others around you as you face each stage of your vision bravely. Because we use our vision to live life at its optimal capacity, as we lose vision, we must use the tools available to harness what vision we have left. Parents will need to encourage their children to use the tools prescribed in order to use as much of their vision as possible. In fact, using the tools available will help the child's brain to continue developing normally. Children do not have to forfeit their mobility, their joy of learning, or human and personal interactions because they are going blind. Children and adults alike with this condition can continue to be mobile and move around their world, learn new things in different contexts, meet friends, fall in love, and build their families.

I finally recognized that I had the good fortune of having a well-rounded life, career, family, and another chance at love. I am rediscovering the man who is the love of my life. Whether sighted or not, isn't that what life is precisely all about—to continue moving forward along life's path despite the challenges. One of the main symptoms of Cone Rod Dystrophy, and the most severe effect, is the eye's reaction to bright light. Rather, it is the inability of the eyes to filter light. The result of the exposure to bright light is extreme discomfort and a reduction of visual acuity. Over time, one may also lose the ability to see colors. These conditions are also referred to as photophobia and achromatopsia, respectively.

Photophobia is characterized by the inability of the photoreceptors in the retina to filter excessive light coming into the eye. When too much light enters the eye, the light causes severe discomfort in the patient. This discomfort can range from mild to extreme. Unprotected patients may even experience severe headaches, migraines, pain in the eyes, disorientation, and disequilibrium. It is common to find that people with this condition squint a lot or are reluctant to go out into bright sunlight. They are even uncomfortable in any situation where light is present. The dimmer the light is, the more comfortable they become. Outdoor activities in the sun are impossible for these patients. Activities in brightly lit spaces such as classrooms or grocery stores are also difficult. Typically, these patients will avoid brightly lit rooms and other bright places. Vitamin D deficiency is of utmost concern for these patients.

One of the commonly prescribed ways of managing photophobia is to use sunglasses designed to reduce glare. This immediately addresses the extreme discomfort the patient experiences. Vision field tests will ultimately reveal the underlying cause of the photophobia. These measures are clearly not a cure for the condition; though, they provide comfort while the investigation is underway. In most cases, the result of the investigation will provide the eye specialist with a plan of action to treat the underlying condition. Photophobia is treatable in cases where the condition is caused by inflammation of the eye or a reaction to medications.

Patients with this condition must make changes to the way they manage their life in order to be comfortable. Most common is to use dim lights at home and avoid situations where there is excessive bright lighting. As can be imagined, just this change will affect vast portions of a person's life and their interactions with others. Just imagine all of the places and situations that are redolent with light in our world, and you understand how drastic a change of lifestyle this will be for Cone Rod Dystrophy patients.

Achromatopsia is also referred to as rod monochromacy, which alludes to the impact on the photoreceptors in the retina. In fact, the cones in the retina are dramatically affected. The patient's retina may not have enough cones, or the cones may be impaired. When there are reduced numbers of cones specifically in the center of the center of the retina, the patient with achromatopsia is typically somewhat or totally color blind. This condition causes several effects; patients are not able to distinguish colors properly and have diminished visual acuity and contrast. Objects will become progressively blurrier with the greatest diminishing impact on distance vision, which becomes extremely poor. Researchers believe that this condition is hereditary; however, it is a rare condition. There is currently no cure for the condition, but patients can manage the symptoms to a certain extent.

Contact lenses and tinted glasses are prescribed in order to provide comfort and increased contrast. Different color shades will offer varying types increased vision, depending on the kind of light present. Patients may need to experiment with different tints to arrive at the best shades possible to maximize his or her vision.

Patients with a severe case of achromatopsia, such as Cone Rod Dystrophy, can only truly find comfort by avoiding bright natural and artificial lights. The ability to monopolize lighting situations will help patients avoid suffering painful headaches and eye pain. In the event that controlling light sources is not possible, patients with severe achromatopsia, and specifically those with Cone Rod Dystrophy, will need frequent downtime in a place with low lighting. One of the curious aspects of Cone Rod Dystrophy is that patients may be able to see much better at night. During the day, however, special glasses, sunglasses, and contact lenses chosen and prescribed by low vision specialists can be used to help filter light and reduce discomfort. In some cases, the low vision specialist and the patient find themselves opening up new ground concerning a rare eye condition. It would be of great help to researchers to connect directly to these cases in order to gather data.

One of my low vision specialists has been working with me for almost ten years. When we first started working together, we had no idea what kind of contact lenses I needed or what shade would be best to try. Although there are a variety of colored lenses, everyone will experience the colors differently. Most patients do well with red-orange lenses. These lenses do a good job of filtering light, and they offer the best contrast. Contrast becomes a big concern for Cone Rod Dystrophy patients. My low vision specialist has been providing me with dark red contact lenses. As we have worked together, and as my vision has changed, she and the specialist that makes the contact lenses have had to be creative in mixing colors that work best for me. Over time, the dark red contact lenses have given way to darker tints, including red/browns. Together, all three of us have learned quite a lot about what tints help me feel most comfortable.

Some of the most important relationships that Cone Rod Dystrophy patients will have will be with professionals in the area of low vision, rehabilitative services, and teachers of the blind and visually impaired. These dedicated people have devoted their lives to making life for the blind a happier and healthier experience. These same individuals work very closely with their patients in solving problems. They have a wealth of information on what may be helpful to patients based on this collaborative experience. It is especially important for parents to develop these relationships to help their visually impaired children. Problems at school will arise because of the child's inability to see whatever teaching aids are being utilized. The teachers may note that the child is struggling, takes longer to do the work, and may have mistakes. These provide clues to the issue of poor vision.

Parents must make it a rule to conference with the teaching team that the child has. For the blind and visually impaired child, the school support team should include vision specialists. The job of school vision specialists is to work with the school district in providing accommodations for the blind and visually impaired child. Their job is also to assist the school in providing the necessary assistive tools to insure that the child is successful in school.

Parents must talk candidly with all of the child's teachers. Although the teachers will be briefed about the physically challenged children in their classrooms, these one-on-one conversations with parents provide teachers with an opportunity to gain more insight into how they can best help the child. Teachers with severely challenged students, and especially vision-impaired students who are mainstreamed, are trained specifically to manage the needs of these children. In the case of children with Cone Rod Dystrophy, because much is still unknown about the condition, teachers will want to gather as much information from the parents as possible. The parents are the experts on what are optimal conditions under which their children will learn best.

Viewing the parents of children with Cone Rod Dystrophy as experts is particularly appropriate. These parents have been engaged, with the help of their vision professionals, in providing an accommodating environment for their child for quite some time. Therefore, the partnership between parents, vision professionals, and the school staff is extremely important, and will last throughout the school years. It is likely that staff members at the child's school will not know much, if anything, about Cone Rod Disorders, so it can be assured that they will welcome the parent's ability to inform them about the disease and how best to manage the symptoms in the classroom.

As most of us know, children generally do not want to appear different from their peers. Because patients with Cone Rod Disorders seem normal, it is of utmost importance to explain some of the known causes, effects, and symptoms of the condition to teachers and school support teams. Parents need to have ideas for teachers on how best to deliver instruction to their child and on how the teachers can respond to queries from other staff members not directly involved. Together, the entire team will have a script that everyone can agree on and utilize. All of these activities truly address accommodation issues. The well-being of the visually impaired child encompasses the need for accommodation safety, self awareness, and self esteem.

One of the very basic conversations to have must be about the importance of lighting. In order to afford the student a level of comfort, avoid disorientation, and improve the student's ability to focus, the student's exposure to bright light must be addressed. As a step one, acknowledgement that the student needs to be comfortable is very important. As previously mentioned, too much exposure to light sources will cause befuddlement, disorientation, headaches, and in some cases vertigo. It cannot be emphasized too much how dramatic an impact this particular aspect to the condition has on the student and the learning process.

For most students, a feeling of comfort and well-being enhances receptivity to the delivery of instruction. Research has shown that children who are well fed, clothed, and happy are more receptive to learning. In addition to these necessary conditions, the visually impaired child must also feel comfortable in the physical learning environment. To feel comfortable in the classroom, the student may need to wear dark glasses throughout the day. Students may also need breaks from the bright classroom during the day. At these times, a dim room set aside for the student is optimal. When using machines with alternate sources of light, such as projectors, televisions, smart boards, computers and other tools, the student may need alternative lesson plans or the instruction delivered in low lighting.

Today's schools can offer students a variety of computerized lessons and other mediums that require bright lights. These modes of instruction enhance the learning opportunities and are enjoyed by students and teachers. Students can learn more through varied delivery experiences. The dedicated and creative teacher will be able to offer these opportunities to the visually challenged student with help from the parent. It is also of great benefit to these students that schools are adept at providing individualized programs to challenged students who are mainstreamed. This gives challenged students the accommodations they need while they are able to interact with their peers.

The Cone Rod Dystrophy student presents interesting challenges to school staff. The student needs low lighting or alternative exercises minimizing light sources, but to do this without causing the child to feel different or to be ostracized. Just wearing dark glasses will shine a spotlight on the student. As the student moves around, seemingly without any trouble, his/her peers may wonder why he or she is wearing dark glasses. While I was teaching, my colleagues would sometimes ask me if I had an accident of some sort and sustained damage to my face. As I found out later, some thought I was being physically abused and hiding black and blue eyes behind my glasses. Yet others thought I even had a drug problem. Heaven only knows what else my colleagues, other staff, and students thought about my wearing dark glasses. I did have a student come up to me one day and say, "You look cool, Miss Vida." I didn't know what else to say except, "Thanks!"

Teachers and school staff can help Cone Rod Dystrophy challenged students by exhibiting appropriate behaviors, and thereby helping by example. Treating the student as they would any other student is preferable to ignoring them or pretending that the student does not have a vision issue. Explaining in simple terms why the student wears dark glasses can be helpful as well. This should be a part of the "script" that has been agreed to by parents. The teacher might just need to say something like, "Sara's eyes are very sensitive to light and needs to protect her eyes," to lay negative perceptions to rest.

When it comes to the delivery of instruction, this condition again poses some challenges. Because almost every object around the student throws off light, the student can become distracted and unfocused. Providing enough contrast for the student in the materials he/she must use can be a helpful strategy. The use of contrast in presenting written material to the Cone Rod Dystrophy student is of utmost importance. To see the lessons well, teachers can practice placing light colors on dark colors to bring into focus work that needs to be done. Dark chalk or markers work best on white or light colors. White on black or black on white materials will work best for students with achromatopsia.

The material covered in this book is directed to the presentation of Cone Rod Dystrophy in school-age children and adults. Although this book focuses on the older child, parents with young children and infants who may have a concern are encouraged to take note of the kinds of toys their young child is attracted to. Parents may notice that their toddler gravitates toward bigger toys or dark-colored ones. Parents may want to ask themselves if the child is forgoing smaller toys, which are age appropriate, in favor of larger ones? Does the child seem not to notice a light-colored toy while it rests on something also light colored? Do they totally ignore or not seem to see small objects? If the answer is consistently yes, then that may be something to discuss with the child's pediatrician. Another interesting item to note is how these toddlers react to meeting new people or interacting with their family members. Do they have trouble figuring out the facial expressions of people around them? Any of these scenarios should prompt parents to discuss what they are noticing with the pediatrician.

As for the older child, a routine screening may alert the parent of the need for more testing to determine the cause of vision loss. Often simple strategies, such as large prints, use of contrasting colors, and experimenting with visual distance, may assist children in the classroom. One of the keys to long-term rehabilitation is to begin eye assessments immediately. There are different types of eye doctors and specialists that may be consulted. These include optometrists, opticians, and ophthalmologists. Once a diagnosis is given, the need to manage the condition so that the individual may continue to live a happy, fulfilled, and productive life requires the services of low vision specialists, rehabilitation specialists, mobility teachers, living skills teachers, and other professionals. It is especially important to learn all that one can about assistive technology and other tools available for the blind and visually impaired.

Low vision rehabilitative, mobility, and living skills services are important for managing the physical manifestation of the condition, as is the managing of the psychosocial and emotional states that are directly affected by having Cone Rod Dystrophy. Many professionals working in the area of psychology, psychiatry, and counseling lend valuable support to individuals facing blindness.

Cone Rod Dystrophy is a term used to refer to a number of disorders that affect the cones and rods in the retina. Therefore, a thorough knowledge of the different manifestations of the condition is advisable. The disorder may be progressive, as is my case. In this situation, the symptoms grow worse over a person's lifetime. The condition may also progress to a point and become stable. Whether the condition continues to cause the cones and rods in the retina to deteriorate, or whether at some point the condition stabilizes, most Cone Rod Dystrophy cases are generally present in childhood.

The primary dysfunction in these cone and rod cells is the progressive nature of the degeneration. This primary feature is what inexorably leads to decreased central visual acuity, severe aversion to bright light, loss of color vision, and night blindness. As the condition progresses, these effects may be followed by loss of peripheral vision, early visual impairment, and blindness. In some cases, there may also be present impairment of other senses such as loss of hearing.

How might a person determine that he or she has a serious retinal problem? What might a person with Cone Rod Dystrophy actually see? This condition is difficult to diagnose for a number of reasons. One of these reasons is that the patient may not perceive a problem with her vision for a great number of years. In fact, many patients routinely visit the eye doctor without any visual problems surfacing.

In my teen years and adulthood, I had regular vision examinations. I was seeing the world around me with very good vision. Although as a preteen, I was diagnosed with astigmatism, and for a time I wore glasses; however, in adulthood, my eye checkups generally indicated twenty-twenty vision. To say that one has twenty-twenty vision is to describe a measurement that the eye doctor does to determine visual acuity. This particular visual measurement means that a person can see small details from twenty feet away in the same way that a person with normal vision can see at the same distance. As a point of reference, a person with twenty-forty vision can see small details from twenty feet away in the same way that a normal person can see those details at forty feet away. I was able to see the smallest detail twenty feet away from me.

I had always checked out as having twenty-twenty vision. Indeed, for a great portion of my life, I had excellent far-vision and good near-vision. It was only much later, and after many visual tests, that I found out that my left eye had always been deficient. I had been conscious of occasionally seeing spots, but the eye doctors reassured me that these were common occurrences. Void of any conclusive tests, the eye doctors did not recommend seeing an ophthalmologist. Meanwhile, my right eye had overcompensated for the weakness in the left eye, so I continued to view the world around me as normal. I never really considered that I had a serious visual problem, and suffice it to say, neither did all of the optometrists I ever visited. Thus, no one noticed the abnormality. It was not until I saw the first floaters in my left eye that I knew something was very wrong with my eyes.

When I was finally diagnosed with Cone Rod Dystrophy, I was seeing floaters and flashes of lights, and had dark spots or scleratomes in my vision. Over the course of two years, I began to notice a change in how I perceived color. One day, I nervously called my ophthalmologist to tell her that I was seeing everything in a sickly shade of green. She gave me an appointment, and after checking my eyes, she counseled me that I was probably going to lose some color vision. I internalized this information and simply asked her if I was going to go totally blind. "Good heavens, no!" she said, "You are going to be able to continue your activities, but you may just have to do them in a different way." The doctor said that I would continue to work, pay bills, and go out socially—everything that I was used to doing.

Her next words set the tone for what would be my new reality. She said, "Now let's talk about assistive technologies available for you so that

49

you can continue to do these things independently". On an emotional level, I found some comfort in her words. They were comforting to me even though intellectually, I knew that I was in for the most dramatic changes of my life. At that time, I did not know all that she meant when she spoke of assistive technologies or how profound a change I would have to make. It was enough that she sounded so confident about my outcomes. It helped me feel confident too.

As it happened, some of what she said turned out to be true—some things not so much. I did learn new strategies to manage daily tasks. I arranged for transportation services to get around and go to work. I learned to use computer software programs designed for the visually impaired and magnification equipment to aid and enhance my work performance. On the other hand, I did lose all ability to see color. As the condition progressed, I had to learn how to cope with some unexpected side effects, such as impaired depth perception and lack of contrast. Over a period of years, I did my research and learned all I could about my condition. Gradually, I felt more knowledgeable, competent, and ultimately, more confident in making decisions surrounding the care and management of my Cone Rod Dystrophy.

Even as I write about my experiences today, I am doing so with the use of computer magnification software on my computer. I also use a large letter keyboard, a CCTV, and handheld magnification tools equipped with cameras. A year ago, I was able to distinguish red, orange, green, and blue from the very far corner of my eyes. Today, I can no longer see them, but I do have functional side vision, but for how long is anyone's guess. One question, however, has been answered to date. What I am absolutely certain of is that there is no central visual acuity. I see the world through a blurry haze that no corrective measures can change.

The loss of color, at the time it was happening, was not a singular event. In other words, it did not happen overnight. It was a gradual loss. After my greening of the world" episode, my vision field changed colors again. I gradually began to see everything in shades of gray and black.

At the time, I would lie in bed at night with the bedside lamp on, and focus on one of the white walls in my bedroom. I tried to concentrate on what I was seeing so that I could describe it to my doctor, hoping to get some answers as to what kind of optical change was occurring. I also kept a written journal in which I described every visual change I was experiencing and how I felt emotionally. The journal writing was therapeutic, but it also provided important anecdotal evidence for determining the course the disease was taking. It did not take me very long to realize that Cone Rod Dystrophy was a condition that was not yet understood in the realm of eye research. The specialists that I was seeing had no real answers.

In fact, what I was reporting to them was furthering their understanding of the problem. As time went on, my doctors were able to read the journal and analyze what changes had taken place. It was exhilarating and disheartening to understand that my doctors were just as baffled by this condition as I was. It continues to be exhilarating because I know that my efforts have helped to advance the research in this area. At the same time, it is disheartening because I recognize that eye research is nowhere near finding a cure or even substantive treatments for Cone Rod Dystrophy.

Describing the primary effects of this condition is one of the tasks I have set for myself in writing this book. I want to describe in detail what I have experienced. As you read these details and effects, be aware that if this is happening to you, it is urgent that you visit an ophthalmologist.

At the same time that my vision was undergoing the previously mentioned color changes, I began to see what is referred to as the "bull's eye" effect in the center of my vision. To describe this effect in simple terms, a very light and opaque circle developed in the very center of my vision. Around that light circle, a dark ring developed. Although the light circle did not appear to change in size, the acuity within this area continued to degenerate. Meanwhile, the dark ring changed size. As I reflect on this today, I realize that the bull's eye in my left eye turned out to be a good predictor of what would eventually happen to my right eye.

Another curiosity I noted with the bull's eye phenomenon was that when I focused on a blank, white wall, I could see what looked like active, wiggling filament-like structures all bunched together in the center of the eye. That bunched up and wriggling mass pervaded the center like a living thing. From time to time, a string-like structure or filament would break loose. It really looked like pieces of the bunch would move away from the center of the eye. Then, as if drawn by a magnet, these pieces would join the mass again. At first, this was frightening to me. These little thread-like structures actually looked like living organisms.

After a while, they simply became a curiosity to me and I studied their behavior. I noted that I could only discern these structures in a darkened room and while focusing on a blank wall. I could bring them into sharp focus by blinking repeatedly. During the day, or in the presence of light, they were not distinguishable. Over time, the bunch dissipated until there were no wriggling filaments left in the center of my eye. Today, I do not see them at all in either eye. As my central acuity diminished, so did this mass of filaments. The day came when they all disappeared and left behind a white space in the center of my eye.

With the passage of time, the bull's eye in my left eye widened and spread. The very center of the eye gradually became blurrier and very white looking. Around that area, the dark ring widened, darkened, and spread. Curiously, while the center of the eye had poor vision, characterized by diminished acuity, I could distinguish objects around me. In the areas of the eye touched by the dark ring, objects could not be seen at all. By shifting my eyes to look up or down, however, the objects would again be distinguishable. In other words, as long as I looked straight ahead, I could see objects in my center of vision, but only very poorly. Likewise, looking straight ahead, nothing beyond the center where the dark ring was present could be seen. However, if I looked up, down, or to my periphery rather than straight ahead, objects could be seen a little better. Today, the bull's eye seems to have become stable. No appreciable change has occurred in the light center or in the wider band of darkness around it.

At about the same time that the bull's eye effect had appeared in my left eye, I also began to experience frequent flashes of light in that eye. The flashes would begin at a point in the outer portion of the eye and circle around the eye until they sputtered away. I thought then that those flashes of light were akin to millions of little flash bulbs flashing at the same time. Another way to describe this effect is like the sputtering that fluorescent lights do before they go on or go out. This particular effect occurred with such frequency that I asked my doctors about it. Every doctor seemed to have a different theory about why it happened. I have asked about this phenomenon many times, but I have yet received what I consider a "good" answer. The fact may be that there really isn't a good answer.

Screening and testing are the first best steps to shedding some light on the symptoms and effects of Cone Rod Dystrophy. The most basic eye test requires that an ophthalmologist look at the retina to make some preliminary determinations. I confess that this test of my vision was always a trial. I felt real distress during these tests due to the lights that the doctors must use for the exam in conjunction with having my eyes dilated. Combined, the bright lights and the dilation were debilitating. Today there is the Optomap—a tool that can test the back of the eye without dilation or using bright lights.

Quite a bit of my anxiety surrounding these tests was due to the fact that my doctors had already told me that there was nothing they could do to fix my eyes. Given this information, I really saw no reason for continuing with annual vision tests. *Why should I have to torture myself each year?* I asked myself. Of course, the dilating and all that bright light was the other cause for my anxiety. I realize now that I was allowing anxiety to overwhelm me. I was willing to give up. The truth is that I needed to continue the vision tests to circumvent any other eye problems that could be treated and to keep learning more about my condition. I needed to learn more so that I could become a better advocate for my family and myself.

In retrospect, I also had a very real fear. I was told I was going blind, and these tests made that event very real. I always feared that I would get a test done and come home incapable of seeing anything. It was a fear of suddenly going totally blind when I was not ready for it to happen. To me, at the time, seeing a little was better than not seeing at all. Consequently, each year I suffered anxiety and panic attacks whenever I had to get my eyes tested with one of those eye-testing machines. Conquering fear sometimes involves letting go of the irrational need for all things to be right. Once I embraced the fact that I was going blind and that I was not helpless, I felt less anxious. Once I conquered my fears, I was able to take tests that graphically showed what was happening in my retina. Some of the tests printed out a picture that showed the bull's-eye effect.

As of this writing, I no longer fear my routine eye tests. I have desensitized myself and have adjusted to the levels of blindness that I have been going through. Most importantly, I've gained a lot of knowledge about the condition that I can now share with others. The bull's eye effect in my right eye has started. There is a lighter central part surrounded by a developing dark ring. The central part of my vision has, as is to be expected, poor acuity. I suspect the same process will take place over time, as described with my left eye.

Although the quality of my vision has gotten progressively worse, I have learned to use whatever residual vision I have to the utmost capacity. As time has gone on, I have adjusted to my degrees of blindness. It is clear that Cone Rod Dystrophy is a condition that renders the person legally blind. There are still many unanswered questions, but that is a reality that patients with this condition must face.

By necessity, I have had to modify the way I do things.

Life in bright light is extremely uncomfortable for Cone Rod Dystrophy patients. Our eyes simply cannot endure the light, as our eyes can no longer filter light. Everything, including objects and people, seems whitewashed when my eyes are unprotected. Without some type of eye filter, I am unable to focus on anything. My eyes wander around, and if I do not put on dark glasses, I am overwhelmed in the presence of light.

In extremely bright circumstances, such as on a bright summer day, I must use dark glasses and dark contact lenses when I am outdoors. Together, they provide the maximum possible filtering so that I can at least go outdoors in some comfort. To be without these kinds of protection, and thus allow myself to be overwhelmed by the presence of light, is to invite blinding headaches, disorientation, and finally debilitation. Yet, I am comfortable as soon as I go into a darker place. I live for dusk. The time when the sun is gone and night has not yet set in is heaven to me. I can take off my dark glasses and let the world see my face.

For some patients with Cone Rod Dystrophy, as it is the case for me, the rods of the eye function poorly. Earlier in the progression of the condition, I was able to see better at night than during the day. Now, I also have trouble seeing at night. Night blindness is a typical symptom of Cone Rod Dystrophy. For me, night blindness means that I can no longer distinguish objects at night with good acuity. Conversely, I need low lighting at night to be able to get around. A curious side effect of Cone Rod Dystrophy is that low lighting at night aids my ability to see, but the same light during the day inhibits my vision.

Although my vision is severely impaired, I can still say that I have a full visual field. That is, with both my eyes open, I see the world all around me, albeit in a hazy, blurred, and unfocused way in shades of black and gray. Even so, I continue to be self-sufficient using the assistive technologies and personal care tools that are available to the visually challenged. I have learned to use a white cane and work with contrast to see things better, among a variety of other helpful strategies.

A perfect example of the use of contrast is when eating out at a restaurant. Generally, at most restaurants, the food is served on a white plate. In this case, patients with Cone Rod Dystrophy are able to locate the food a little easier. A person may not be able to tell what he is eating or whether the meat is to the right or the left of the plate, but at least the food can be seen. The patient will register the dark food against the white plate. The food will definitely be seen much better on a white plate than on a dark one.

I have been in restaurants where the plates are dark and therefore offer no contrast. In such cases, I simply ask that the food be placed on a white or light-colored plate. It is good to view your plate as if it is the face of a clock—practice placing your food at twelve o'clock, three o'clock, six o'clock, and nine o'clock. For example, place your vegetables at twelve, your meat at three, your bread at six, and your side dish at nine, or whatever order works best for you. Dinner companions can also be helpful by telling you where the food is located on the plate. The restaurant may even be happy to exchange your plate for a lighter colored one if you ask. Learning simple strategies for daily living will make life more comfortable and much easier to manage. Once you learn some simple strategies and become skilled at these, you can be free to be yourself and have enjoyable interactions with people and things around you.

One of many lessons I have learned is that once I accepted my Cone Rod Dystrophy, I began to rely less on seeing and more on using my mind and my other senses. It is not in my opinion that my other senses somehow become superior or super human—I have just learned to use them more efficiently. You may have heard others say that in a blind person, other senses become more developed and essentially compensate for the loss of vision. I do not believe this to be the case. My sense of hearing has not become dramatically keener because I am going blind. I have simply learned to use my other senses more effectively.

Because I am not relying on sight to give me the clues I need to manage the world around me, I can now hear all the clues that I have been missing, due to my dependence on hearing. Before I became blind, I crossed a street by waiting for the pedestrian light to show me when to cross over. Now I listen for the flow of traffic to tell me when it is safe to cross. This is a learned, focused, and skilled way to manage daily living. After investing the time, effort, and perseverance that one must have in order to understand the condition, it is time to gain needed skills.

The next step is to learn different strategies for completing tasks, which lead to a variety of skills that make life easier to manage and more enjoyable. As one comes to terms with one's blindness, there is less reliance on visual cues and more on the mind, senses, strategies, and skills.

Indeed, being a Cone Rod Dystrophy patient has advantages and disadvantages. This dichotomy is evident in regards to the use of one's other senses. Specifically, Cone Rod Dystrophy patients may have some residual vision for a great part of their life. They are able to continue to use whatever vision they may have to its utmost capacity, especially with aids such as magnification tools. Therefore, as uncomfortable as it may be, reacting to visual cues is still within the realm of possibility for many Cone Rod Dystrophy patients. One cannot always distinguish a duck from a fire hydrant, as one woman put it, yet patients are able to distinguish that something is there and avoid stumbling into it.

It is something of a miracle and a trial to have this ability. It allows one to see some things fairly well and other things not at all. Friends and family may consider whether you are becoming loony. Yet, for those with Cone Rod Dystrophy, the worlds of reality and illusion merge. It would be of value to have more studies about how these two worlds collide. One poignant example of this miracle or curse happened to me during the tragedy of 9/11. Sadly, I could not see with clarity what was happening to the twin towers, but I discerned enough to experience the magnitude of that tragic day.

When someone is working on our roof, I know where the worker is located on the roof from the worker's speech and sounds, and I am able to judge the height. I can tell what is very high up and what is low through my hearing. Yet, I cannot tell what the worker is actually doing, wearing, or even what he or she looks like.

If I hear two dogs barking in the neighborhood, they may both sound like Chihuahuas with high-pitched *yips*, but I am able to determine if one is larger than the other. However, if a large dog is sitting silently next to a fire hydrant, the two are indistinguishable from each other.

I remember sauntering confidently up my front walkway to the front door one fine summer day. I looked down to see a stick lying on the front step. I hunched down and picked up the stick to throw it into the hedges. Imagine my surprise when that stick wriggled and wrapped itself around my wrist. I had picked up a little snake that had been out sunning itself on our front stoop. Fortunately, it was only a garden-variety little snake. I haven't picked up anything from the ground again.

The fact that one has some residual vision may be advantageous at the onset. As the condition progresses, however, as most of the cases do, visual cues become increasingly distorted and not to be trusted. By necessity, one relies more so on other senses. The other senses seem more pronounced because a person already has an orientation as to the things in the world. In the blind or visually challenged person, these senses enhance what the individual already knows. Thus, the teaching modes, assistive technologies, mobility training, and other necessary strategies and skills that must be learned may be hampered or enhanced by context.

Turning back to the issue of eye exams, I now can face my eye exam each year with confidence. I know that I can have my eyes dilated, look into flashing cameras, and receive ERGs and whatever else has to be done. I know that I will return home the same as I left it. Furthermore, it is important to have these tests in order to catch any other problems that may surface. Problems such as cataracts, glaucoma, or macular degeneration are treatable.

It is important to remember, especially as one ages, that other conditions will likely arise. Cone Rod Dystrophy may be the least of my worries in a world that includes high blood pressure/hypertension, diabetes, and cancer. Yet, by no means are we to succumb to worrying about what could happen. Life is to be lived. It is helpful for me to remember that I am going blind, but I'm not losing my mind. Rational thinking is a sure way to conquer irrational fears. Thus, a necessary first step, and a most rational decision to make, is to set up an eye exam. The next step is to do determine the best eye professional for helping your vision if you are seeing spots, floaters, and flashes.

CHAPTER 3:
GATHERING KNOWLEDGE

Differences among eye doctors and specialists

In our daily lives, we accept the concepts of routine overhauls, maintenance, assessments, analysis, and evaluations. From keeping our homes and cars in tiptop shape to exploring the depths of our commitment to friends, loved ones, our country, and ourselves, we submit to surveys and assessments on a routine basis. This is why we have annual exams of all kinds. We want to ensure that we are working at utmost capacity.

When systems fail, we feel powerless, disoriented, unbalanced, confused, overwhelmed, and depressed. We come face to face with the realization that our lives are fragile, unpredictable, and sometimes chaotic. We realize that the things we rely on to make us happy are finite.

To solve our problems, we may have meetings, convene commissions, or have summits. If we can get some answers, we can fix the problem— all will be well, and we can continue on our way. We follow this practice in most facets of our lives. We take our cars to the automotive center for diagnostic tests, our psyches to a therapist, our faltering relationships to family counselors, and our bodies to medical doctors.

We expect that given an exam and some tests, we will know what to do so that all ends well. Similarly, we convince ourselves that a diagnostic test will tell us what is going wrong with our health and how to correct the problem. It is a good practice to visit medical doctors to find out what could be going wrong, but we will not always receive the answers we expect.

In the United States, we spend extraordinary amounts of money to get the best health care possible. The access to care is expensive and not within reach of every citizen. Yet, those who have health care expect to have good health. When a physical ailment, disease, or life-altering condition appears in our lives, we must remind ourselves that everything does not always end the way we expect it to.

Facing a yet unspecified illness or condition, the appropriate response is to schedule a diagnostic evaluation and medical tests. Most of us visit the medical doctor, dentist, and eye doctor on an annual basis. If one is fortunate enough to have good, accessible, and affordable health care, the difference between prevention and cure is early intervention.

When something is not quite right with your health, an assessment is the first step. However, this by itself is not enough to move you forward on the path to wellness. One's personal outlook and attitude is just as important. We may well acknowledge that medical doctors may not be able to offer all of the answers. Quite often, no answers, magic pills, or ointments, and sometimes not even surgery will correct the problem. At such times, we seek the best solution we can in order to live as happy and productive a life as possible. A positive, optimistic outlook towards the future, despite the hardships that may lie ahead, will get a person through many of life's challenges.

The support that you may receive from family, friends, and other support systems is invaluable in helping you get through the tough spots. We want to be happy, and we can be happy. Happiness is achievable, especially when we know as much as we can about our conditions. Learning strategies and skills to manage them efficiently gives us the tools to live a happy and productive life.

Blindness due to Cone Rod Dystrophy is a life altering and overwhelming event. How to face going blind and loving life despite it requires all of the inner strength one can muster. On a daily basis, those of us who are going blind must face it as courageously as we can.

The first step is to be brave each day. The second step is to learn as much as possible about the condition. The third step is to manage the condition by learning the necessary strategies and skills for coping on an ongoing basis. The fourth step is to utilize your internal and external support systems to bolster your spirit and your faith so that you can live happily.

The same is true concerning children or the elderly. Those who care for them must pay close attention to what they are saying that can and cannot see. Their caretakers must be observant of how they are relating visually to the world around them.

The type of eye condition determines the kind of doctor needed. A lot depends on the eye problem that the patient is experiencing. Typically, most people visit their optometrist for annual checkups. The primary job of optometrists is to diagnose and treat vision problems, eye diseases, and related visual conditions. They prescribe eyeglasses, contact lenses, and medications to treat eye disorders. When a condition requires surgery, they cannot perform them. They can provide before and after surgical care, but they must refer the patient to a specialist.

An optician works alongside an optometrist or an eye surgeon in a supportive role. When a patient's case is outside of the purview of the optometrist, he or she will refer the patient to an ophthalmologist for further care. In such cases, the need is evident for specialized tests and a different diagnosis and treatment of the eye condition, as it is beyond the jurisdiction of the optometrist.

Ophthalmologists are eye doctors that specialize in the medical and surgical care of the eyes, eye disease, and injuries. An ophthalmologist is qualified to deliver total eye care and vision services, eye exams, medical and surgical eye care, and the diagnosis and treatment of disease and visual complications caused by other conditions such as diabetes. Once it has been established that the patient has a condition that requires specialized treatments and assistive technologies, a low vision specialist is consulted.

Low vision specialists are visual care professionals that work with patients who have reduced vision or are legally blind. These are patients with visual impairments, some of which may lead to total blindness. The low vision specialist works in a supportive role to aid optometrists and eye surgeons in delivering care. In most cases, these patients are unable to use prescribed corrective lenses, and thus the low vision specialist works to provide the most appropriate tools and technologies available to help the patient make the most of the vision they have.

With the help of optometrists, opticians, ophthalmologists, and low vision specialists, I achieved a proper diagnosis, the best prognosis possible, appropriate glasses, contact lenses, and low vision tools to help me function in daily living and be productive at work. Once the patient is diagnosed as legally blind, low vision specialists are able to file the paperwork necessary for the patient to be considered disabled by state and federal government agencies.

In the United States, when your vision cannot be corrected with lenses better than twenty-twenty in your good eye, or you have lost peripheral vision, you are eligible for the disability classification.

For quite some time, the World Health Organization has reported an increasing number of people at risk for visual impairment. As the world populations grow and age, demographic data suggest growing numbers of people affected by blindness. Potentially on the rise are eye impairments and conditions leading to blindness, such as age-related macular degeneration or AMD, diabetic retinopathy, and glaucoma.

Globally, according to the World Health Organization, more than 161 million people were visually impaired in 2002, of whom 124 million people had low vision and thirty-seven million were blind. Given local and regional data on visual issues, we can deduce that worldwide, there are wide variations in reported numbers. Conceivably, some areas have higher numbers of certain types of visual issues as compared to other regions. Regardless of these variations, the concern remains. As the world population grows and ages, so does the risk for visual related issues. It is truly a part of our human condition.

CHAPTER 4:
TAKING CONTROL

*Differences among eye tests, diagnoses,
prognoses, and treatment options*

My journey towards understanding my eye problem began at one of the best vision centers in the country, the Georgetown Center for Sight. At this facility, I was under the care of an eminent, well-known specialist and one of the pioneers in Cone Rod Dystrophy research, Dr. Georgia Chrousos. She and I embarked on what was a five-year journey toward the day when she said, "I know what this is!"

Our work began with a series of visual acuity tests, which screen for how clearly one can see. Those who have access to vision care visit an eye doctor for an annual checkup and experience a visual test. Typically, the individual is asked to read letters from an eye chart while seated at a distance from the chart. In patients with Cone Rod Dystrophy, the distance at which letters on an eye chart can be seen decreases over time.

Patients with serious retinal complaints are also given color vision acuity tests. These tests are used in the screening for Cone Rod Dystrophy, and they show how clearly and accurately the patient sees colors. There are many variations of these tests. The color vision test I remember most vividly from my testing at the Georgetown Center for Sight, the Wilmer Eye Institute at Johns Hopkins, and at the National Institutes for Health involved presenting to the patient color images containing hidden numbers. Invariably, Cone Rod Dystrophy patients have trouble recognizing the numbers.

In tests where recognition of colors is being examined, Cone Rod Dystrophy patients tend to have poor results. A curious feature of this condition is that many patients may not readily see colors when looking directly at them. Instead, patients may be able to see the colors with their peripheral vision. During my tenure as a secondary school teacher, many of my colleagues were perplexed by my ability to sometimes see things and at other times not see them. There were times when I could not recognize colleagues familiar to me or even recognize a friend. A Cone Rod Dystrophy patient might hear that a friend or colleague is angry with her. The conversation between them might go something like, "I thought you were upset with me," the friend says.

"Why would you think that?" the patient answers.

"Because you passed right by me this morning; I waved to you, but you didn't even smile back!" the slighted friend responds.

Many of my friends and colleagues, and even some of my family members thought that I was faking my blindness because they saw me performing my tasks perfectly well. A Cone Rod Dystrophy patient seems to blend seamlessly into what is considered normal visual behavior. This ability can be helpful and a hindrance. In the workplace, a Cone Rod Dystrophy worker strives to demonstrate her productivity. As a parent, friend, lover, or any of the other roles the person plays in her life, she wants to be like those who are sighted. The visually challenged individual will be focused on making daily tasks, relationships, interactions, and other facets of life continue just as those with normal vision do. The patient will try to convince herself and others that she is a self-sufficient, functioning, and a productive member of the community.

At times, this ability to overcompensate visual impairment can be a hindrance. When a Cone Rod Dystrophy patient needs accommodations at work or in school, such as assistive technologies or any other kind of aid, the patient must prove that she is indeed visually challenged.

Individuals with Cone Rod Dystrophy may sometimes feel emotionally conflicted. On the one hand, they want to be seen as competent and able to perform tasks in the same way as those who are sighted. For some, behaving as if they have normal vision may mean being perceived as self-sufficient, self-reliant, independent, productive, and efficient members of society. Yet, to be visually challenged may also imply that there are times when the individual requires specialized conditions. These are needed for the majority of visually challenged persons in order for them to perform at their best ability. These specialized conditions require appropriate accommodations. In this way, the visually challenged individual can perform at a level equal to peers doing the same tasks.

In the field of education, a popular cliché is that every challenge is an opportunity. I believe that every challenge is a challenge. Accepting, understanding, managing, and solving the challenges we face helps us to create a nurturing environment in which opportunities can grow. We must also recognize the differences among various opportunities that cross our paths. Some will lead to positive outcomes. Some will only lead to more difficulties. When appropriate accommodations are made in the work environment for a physically challenged individual, challenges are overcome, opportunities to progress are nurtured, and positive outcomes are possible.

As the condition progresses further, the visually challenged individual, as well as others concerned, must recognize that there will be limitations. The person will need appropriate accommodations designed to address these specific limitations. Addressing these needs will help to keep a valued employee in the workplace. What is not wanted or needed by anyone with a disability is pity. Just because the individual is visually challenged does not mean that he or she is somehow lessened due to needing accommodations.

Most visually challenged individuals of working age want to be perceived as having the same capability as their counterparts. Understanding these extremely emotional concepts can occasionally be an exhausting challenge. The lessons learned from this exercise, however, are well worth the effort. For a visually challenged person, understanding these conflicting ideas, feelings, and emotions and coming to terms with them may help to lighten the spirit.

Typically, Cone Rod Dystrophy patients have trouble seeing the light as it moves to the center. Some Cone Rod Dystrophy patients may have trouble seeing the blinking lights due to "blind spots" in their visual field, called scleratomas.

The objective of these visual field testing machines is to produce a diagram of all the areas in your field of vision that you can see and not see. This diagram is useful to ophthalmologists in their discussions with their patients. This test also reveals what the eye physically looks like.

An ERG test or electroretinogram is one of the first tests ordered for the screening of a visual problem, especially for those patients who may have a retinal disorder such as Cone Rod Dystrophy. This test actually looks at the functioning of the cones and rods in the retina. One word of caution: these tests are costly. The cost may be manageable for those with health insurance or access to vision care. I was fortunate to have health insurance, which allowed me to go to the Georgetown Center for Sight and receive extremely good vision care.

The ERG test is only done in a small number of centers around the United States. It is only used when all other tests are unable to confirm a diagnosis of a retinal disorder. The patient's eyes are numbed with special drops, and a special kind of contact lens is placed in each eye. This lens is attached to electrodes that determine how the cones and rods are functioning. The test is first conducted in a dark room to measure the function of the rods and then in a lighted room to measure the cones. Flashes of light are administered in order to stimulate the retina and activate the function of the cones and rods. The electrical responses are recorded. This test can confirm a diagnosis of Cone Rod Dystrophy since the recordings of the electrical impulses will show a dysfunction of the cones and rods.

The most important vision test, and which in my case led to my ophthalmologist's epiphany about my diagnosis, is the fundus photograph. A special camera takes a photograph of the back of the eye and retina. The eyes are dilated, and once the photograph is taken, the doctor can make a convincing determination. Many other tests are at the disposal of the doctor. An eye specialist might order other tests with the objective of eliminating the possibility of other disorders.

In addition to the aforementioned tests, my eye specialist at the Georgetown Center for Sight also ordered blood tests, an MRI, and an EKG. Blood tests can determine underlying causes such as viral/bacterial infections or conditions such as Lyme disease. An EKG, or electrocardiogram, can determine whether there is an underlying heart condition or if there are problems with other internal organs.

The MRI or Magnetic Resonance Imaging scan is a tool used in radiology. This technique uses a magnetic process, radio waves, and a computer to produce images of tissues and structures in the body. The MRI scanner produces very detailed images with high resolution. The MRI scan can detect tiny changes of structures within the body. The images it produces can help a medical professional accurately detect disease or trauma in the body.

The MRI scan is an extremely accurate way of detecting trauma to the brain as evidenced by bleeding or swelling of the brain. Eye specialists will order this test for patients who have had aneurysms, strokes, tumors, or other abnormalities of the brain.

Vision testing is therefore useful and necessary, and it can be prolonged. At times, patients can feel uncomfortable about the number of tests they are taking, feel that the tests are useless or offer conflicting diagnosis, or they can feel despondent about what the tests are showing. Yet, when working together as a team in a trusting and honest relationship, a patient and doctor can reach a successful diagnosis.

To help this wellness-driven partnership to grow and function takes effort on the part of the patient and the doctor. It is important for the patient to be aware of what he is experiencing, and to be able to acknowledge it and discuss it with his doctor. The doctor's willingness to be open and frank with the patient is vital for finding the right diagnosis, treatment, and prognosis. The doctor must be willing to invest time and effort with the patient to get to this level of honesty. Getting to know the patient is a prelude to the difficult conversations that will come later on. The doctor-patient relationship, as with any relationship, can only be as strong as what each party brings to it. If the hard work of establishing this rapport takes place, the more difficult explanations that the doctor must make later on in the patient's treatment will be done on fertile ground. The patient will trust what the doctor says and feel that he or she has been an active participant in the process.

The English poet William Ernest Henley (1849-1903) wrote a powerful poem that has been quoted by many people through the years, whether for good purposes or ill. In the poem titled "Invictus," his words resonate just as strikingly today as they did when he wrote them. Each verse in this poem speaks to the indomitable nature of the human spirit. The first verse, however, has always called out to me:

Out of the night that covers me,
Black as the Pit from pole to pole
I thank whatever gods may be
For my unconquerable soul.

This poem speaks to me so powerfully because it tells us that we can conquer our shortcomings and our fears. We have to remember that the study of retinal disorders is still in its infancy. Eye care specialists are learning more each day as they research eye disorders. Each time they have the opportunity to work with a patient with a retinal disorder, they add to the body of knowledge in the field. I look at it as a privilege and a responsibility to share my experiences with my eye specialists. It is a way that I can contribute to ongoing research, find solace for myself, and help others in the process. The work that doctors such as Dr. Georgia Chrousos and others are doing is paving the way to groundbreaking research and eventual substantive treatments in the future.

Learning to face the adversities in our lives is a lifelong, everlasting skill. Courage in the face of adversity is a necessary element to overcoming life's challenges. This is not a new or earth-shattering revelation. People all over the world face the troubles in their lives with awesome courage every day. Those battling illnesses, personal tragedies, and national disasters are real life examples of courage in the face of incomprehensible tragedy. In my case, my family has been my role model. Both my children have faced difficult challenges with courage and a generosity of spirit. They help me face what fears I have along my journey into blindness through their example.

None of us is born courageous. I believe we acquire it along life's pathways through practice, just as we do other skills. Courage is that which allows infants to take their first steps into an unknown, exciting world. It accompanies the soldier into what may be his or her final steps on earth. It is what motivates people to overcome natural disasters and rebuild their lives again.

As the elation of finally being given an accurate diagnosis subsided, the time had come to have a discussion with my eye specialist. Armed with knowledge about my condition, we had to discuss my prognosis for the future, the treatments available to me, and most importantly, how my life would be impacted by the eye condition. Dr. Chrousos had to find a way to tell me that there was no cure for Cone Rod Dystrophy, and that I was going to be legally blind. I am convinced that doctors struggle emotionally when delivering such news to a patient. There is no easy way to break news such as this. Like any other life altering diagnosis, the way in which the doctor delivers the news and the patient reacts will be a testament to the kind of doctor-patient relationship that has been forged over the months of testing and discovery. That both the patient and doctor will be deeply affected by this moment is unavoidable.

A contentious relationship between patient and doctor throughout this journey of discovery can only lead to a fractious, hurtful, and conflicted moment of revelation. Thankfully, my eye specialist and I had developed an honest relationship. She and I had worked and learned together as we progressed through the various stages of establishing the diagnosis. Therefore, I had a doctor who I trusted to tell me the truth and to help me figure out what the next steps would be in my treatment.

In the case of patients with Cone Rod Dystrophy, there is no medical next step. There is no cure for this condition. The next step in the process moves quickly to the management stage.

Sometimes the doctor-patient relationship has another profound moment. That is when the relationship comes to an end by necessity. My eye specialist started me on a path and another process that would consume the rest of my life—she helped me understand more about my eye condition and managing its effects.

One can't simply say goodbye or adequately show one's deep appreciation for a person who has been such an integral part of one's life. I cannot express my deep appreciation for the able assistance, compassionate support, and simple human comfort that Dr. Chrousos gave to me.

Regrettably, when a few years later I went back to the Georgetown Center for Sight to thank Dr. Chrousos for all she had done on my behalf, I found that she had gone back to her native Greece to continue her wondrous work. This book is my tribute to her, and to all the eye professionals who have worked with me along this journey, and to all of those doctors and researchers continuing in the struggle to find answers.

The next step in my journey began with my introduction to low vision specialists. These specialists helped me acquire hand-held magnifiers, special tinted glasses, specially tinted contact lenses, and other optical aids. They allowed me to try out these optical aids in their offices so that I could choose the ones that worked best for me. Low vision specialists are invaluable as the first step towards freedom from dependency.

These eye professionals brought perspective and the sense of reality to just how Cone Rod Dystrophy was affecting my vision.

With the aid of low vision specialists, Cone Rod Dystrophy patients are able to maximize whatever vision they have. This is done with optical aids such as magnifiers, computer magnification programs, and a closed circuit television apparatus (CCTV). These tools help patients complete the necessary tasks of daily living.

Another key partner in the process of working with low vision specialists is the federal, state, and local Departments of the Blind and Vision Impaired. These departments enable access to many assistive programs for instruction in mobility, daily living, and personal care. These agencies provide programs to guide the blind and visually impaired toward self-reliance and self-sufficiency. They provide funds for purchasing tools and equipment that will be helpful in the individual's training. They allow individuals to continue to be productive and effective in their workplace.

Most importantly, however, these agencies provide the funds needed to buy equipment and optical tools for their clients, as well as to pay for the services of eye care professionals. Through the Department of the Blind and Vision Impaired in my state, I worked with professionals knowledgeable in computer hardware and software programs. My goal was to continue to be a productive worker and member of society. The counselors understood my goals and developed a strategy for helping me to attain them. Using the equipment at their offices, I was taught how to use the machines that would be appropriate for my needs. There is where I was introduced to the diverse computer programs available, hand-held tools, and CCTVs.

Working with the counselors, I also learned more about how my condition works with different types of tools and what techniques I could use to maximize my visual ability. The agency's staff is trained not only to work with clients at their office, but they can also order the equipment that the client is eligible to receive. The staff will also deliver the equipment to your workplace or home. Once there, the staff will install the equipment, set it up to the specifications already worked out with you during training, and follow up with you later.

These agencies also employ teachers of the blind and visually impaired. Their job is to teach and train individuals in strategies and skills for living and doing daily tasks. These professionals and teachers are invaluable in helping a blind or visually impaired learner come to terms with blindness. The teachers are often physically challenged as well. They are able to understand and relate more keenly to what the learner is experiencing. In fact, they often use these same tools in their daily lives. I have great admiration for these low vision specialists, mobility instructors, daily living teachers, and equipment trainers. This book is also my tribute to them because they have the task of guiding and assisting me toward self-reliance and the preservation of my independence.

In summary, the main action that someone experiencing vision problems is encouraged to take is to set up an appointment with an optometrist or ophthalmologist for a vision checkup as soon as possible. An assessment by an optometrist or ophthalmologist specializing in vision challenges is a priority when a vision problem surfaces. These professionals will be able to offer the information needed about possible vision problems, conditions, or disorders. They will administer many tests in order to find the underlying cause of the vision problem and to determine a diagnosis. Among the tests that the eye specialist might order are blood analysis, visual field tests, neurological exams, an MRI, and an ERG. Very often, a doctor may go through several possible reasons for the condition before he or she arrives at the correct diagnosis.

This process may take a very long time and test the limits of your patience and endurance. It is very important to have a trusting relationship with the vision care specialists. Thus, there needs to be mutual respect, honesty, truth, and trust between the patient and doctor. The patient is responsible for inquiring about the tests, treatments, and services he will be receiving. The more information the patient has, the better he will be able to make appropriate decisions about his care. The patient ought not to be afraid to ask questions. Important to one's self-advocacy is a willingness to do research regarding one's visual problem. The Internet, other patients, and support groups in the community are places to start the research.

The greater part of the information gathered, however, will come from the eye specialist. It is the doctor's responsibility to educate the patient about his or her condition, do the appropriate vision tests, and rule out all the possible problems causing the condition in order to zero in on the definite cause. In short, the doctor must deliver a diagnosis. Further, the doctor will want to explore the medical or surgical remedies available to the patient. The patient and doctor must establish a plausible course of action together. In cases where treatment is warranted, the doctor orders a prescription or treatment for the problem. In my mind, the greatest moral responsibility that the doctor has is to inform the patient of all the options, or lack thereof. Whether the condition is treatable with optical aids, medications, or surgeries, or whether it cannot be treated conventionally—the patient needs to know.

A word of caution is appropriate here. The patient may not always experience a moment when all of the testing pieces come together tidily to produce a diagnosis. In many cases, the condition cannot be identified. This kind of situation is understandably frustrating. It can leave the patient and doctor in a quandary as to how to proceed in alleviating the effects of the condition. A trying period of trial and error may ensue. It is precisely in these situations that a strong doctor-patient relationship, loving support from significant others, and faith and courage within oneself can help to sustain the patient.

The "ah-ha" moment for me was when my ophthalmologist used a camera to take pictures of my retina. This was the moment when she could say with certainty, "Oh yes, that's what it is! You have Cone Rod Dystrophy!" This was a moment of determination and elation for both of us. After five years of searching for an answer, there was heartfelt satisfaction in being able to find a reason for what was happening to me. Now, we were able to enter the rehabilitation phase. This phase started with my doctor's explanation of my visual impairment, how I might have come by it, and what could be done about it.

This moment affected me very deeply. On one hand, I felt a sense of relief that we had finally come to the end of the testing stage. It had taken a long time and a lot of energy to get to this point. I had gone through an emotional upheaval with which I was still trying to come to terms. I appreciated my doctor's honesty and her support when I was besieged by doubts and fears. I trusted in her competency, and therefore in the information that she gave me on the nature of my condition. When it came to my prognosis, it was also time to come to terms with the truth.

For me, it was very important to hear the truth from my doctor. Although overwhelming, the truth allowed me to take the first decisive steps on my own toward my future. Not getting all of the truth from a doctor can violate the trust that has been so painstakingly developed and nurtured. Moreover, withholding the truth slows the progress that the patient needs to make physically, psychologically, and emotionally. I had the most startling realization upon receiving the diagnosis that I had Cone Rod Dystrophy. Not only was I going blind, but I also had been going blind for quite some time. That day was not the first day of losing my vision; it was the first day that I began living with blindness.

This knowledge was like a sudden emotional earthquake that shook my world to its foundation. A sense of helplessness overwhelmed me when I was told that the condition was progressive and untreatable. I was shocked to learn that there is no cure for Cone Rod Dystrophy and that doctors do not know what happens as the individual grows older. Although loss of central acuity and peripheral vision is a given, my doctor could not say with all certainty if there would be total blindness in my future.

For that fateful moment, the feelings of desolation, aloneness, and doom were complete. Anyone who can imagine receiving a diagnosis of severe or terminal illness can relate to these feelings. In fact, we have all felt the same feelings of trepidation at some point in our lives. These feelings may come in varying degrees, but they do come. When they do, we can succumb to them or we can weather them.

Yet, this degree of openness, frankness, honesty, and truth is essential. Only in this context can the patient move forward. At this moment, I felt that this disease had circumvented the goals I had set for my family, my relationships, and my entire life. It felt as if it was a blight on my very soul.

I left the doctor's office and went out into the fading light of a late afternoon in the fall. I looked around me and thought that I could already sense what the world would eventually look like for me all the time. I began to understand that everything around me would eventually blur and fade to gray—perhaps to black. I stood there for a long time taking in the day as the sun was setting and the shadows lengthened from dusk into the early evening. The realization fell over me as I drove home. One day, I would no longer drive—I was going to be blind.

Months passed by where I went through my daily routines feeling numb. I had two children to take care of, my career as a teacher, and other duties and responsibilities just like everyone else. I vowed to take it a day at a time for as long as I could. It took some time for me to realize that I did not have to abandon my goals or any other part of my life; I simply had to approach them in another way. I learned to look toward a future that could still be very bright. I just needed to accept the help that was available.

For a patient suffering vision loss, once the prognosis has been made, the ophthalmologist must focus on how to help the patient adjust to the unwanted news. The doctor will help the patient understand and accept the challenges ahead and plan for future successes. There is still hope despite one's blindness. The doctor's other responsibility is to put the patient into contact with the professionals and programs available.

These will aid the patient in learning how to live with the vision he or she will have.

The doctor will also do what he or she can to support the patient emotionally. I believe that a strong support system, one that includes family, friends, significant others and colleagues, along with the professionals that will be involved in the patient's life, is extremely important in the overall well-being of the patient. For this reason, part of the closure discussion that the doctor has with the patient is how to build up these relationships.

In this manner, the phase consisting of the discovery of the eye problem and the subsequent discovery of the condition through testing, diagnosis, prognosis, and planned treatment program comes to an end. Certain eye problems can be medically treated, in which case the doctor-patient relationship may continue. In the case of Cone Rod Dystrophy, however, there is no medical treatment currently available, so the patient moves on to the management phase of the condition.

Understanding the nature of the condition, as previously mentioned, begins with gathering as much information as possible. This is as important as learning about the support and assistance available through the various programs within the community. Learning to live with and manage Cone Rod Dystrophy requires the patient to gain essential knowledge, which will aid in the emotional and psychosocial adjustment of the patient.

The individual's family and loved ones should also be educated on the condition. To confront this new reality, the patient needs a variety of support systems. For those who are still a part of the workforce, it is of paramount importance to learn about the Americans with Disabilities Act regulations, laws, and norms regarding workplace accommodations. Adjustments and accommodations will need to be made as loss of vision becomes more pronounced. Likewise, in the educational setting, appropriate accommodations will have to be considered.

The adaptation of alternative and optical aids is the primary concern in the management phase of this disease. The majority of visually impaired people can be helped by these aids in order to make the most of the vision they still have. For the blind and visually impaired, there are large print books, books in Braille, audiobooks, magnification machines (CCTVs), and computer programs. The computer programs offer magnification of text and allow the text to be read audibly. New technologies are coming into being on an ongoing basis, and low vision specialists are the key people with whom to interact regarding these.

According to much of the latest research in the field of vision care, there is an increase in the number of people with visual impairments. Eye conditions that lead to blindness such as age-related macular degeneration, diabetic retinopathy, and glaucoma are increasing. Treatments for the various conditions are costly and out of reach for many. Alternative and optical aids are very expensive, and most people cannot afford them. Accessibility and affordability are increasingly important to large segments of the affected population. Most states offer assistance with the increasing costs associated with visual assessments, treatments, and purchase of appropriate visual aids and equipment. In addition, through the federal government, programs for the blind and vision impaired are available as well. Nevertheless, more programs for the blind and vision impaired will be needed as research continues to reveal new information and treatments.

It is important for individuals with vision problems to become knowledgeable about the programs available through organizations in their community and through the government at the state and federal level. For some individuals, another important step in their evolution as a person living with blindness or vision impairment may be to become an advocate for him or herself and others. Becoming involved in lobbying efforts, peer outreach, mentoring, coaching, and other areas of advocacy can be of tremendous psychological, emotional, and social fulfillment.

Lobbying is an example of an essential area of advocacy. A sustained effort to lobby local, state, and federal government agencies, as well as private institutions, continues to be indispensable. Historically, lobbying by ordinary citizens struggling to manage vision impairment and blindness issues has been instrumental in establishing programs to help individuals, especially low income/uninsured patients. Organizations providing critical services to this population have provide the necessary vehicle for joining the voices of those affected. Through their focused commitment to bringing these voices to the appropriate levels of government, major pieces of legislation have been made into law, and this effort continues today. Specifically, more attention has been focused on the high cost of vision care and the inability of low income and uninsured patients to receive the proper care. Due to the emphasis on this issue of high cost adversely affecting accessibility for many people, other barriers to this population have also surfaced. Transportation services, alternative optical aids, and access to participation in ongoing research are other areas that are inaccessible to low income and uninsured individuals with vision problems.

CHAPTER 5:
THIS IS YOUR MOMENT

Living with blindness and managing lifestyle changes

There is nothing like bumping into glass doors to help one realize that lifestyle changes need to be made. I recall having a luncheon date with friends at a very nice restaurant. I was looking forward to meeting my friends, and so I took a cab to the restaurant. I got out of the cab right in front of the entrance. I bounded out of the cab with vigor and confidence and walked right into their highly polished glass double doors. I thought I saw an open entryway. I suffered the embarrassment of having everyone inside the restaurant witness my faux pas. Sometimes it pays to put your hand out and make sure that you are not walking into a glass door. Had I been going to the restaurant at night, I would have had a better chance of getting it right.

Another opportunity presented itself to me when my daughter and I were leaving her orthodontist's office. We were going down the steps in the front of the office when I mistook the last step for the level landing. Fortunately, my daughter was there to help me avoid a bad spill. Her first words were, "Where is your cane, Mom?" Of course, it was back at the house. As they say, pride goes before a fall—literally. I have learned to set aside prideful thoughts in favor of safety.

For me, living with blindness is as complex as living with in-laws. A number of implications, adjustments, and compromises must be made on a daily basis. When living with in-laws, one's lifestyle is affected by the need to create a harmonious home environment for everyone. Success is determined by the flexibility that everyone demonstrates in daily routines. As anyone who has lived in this situation knows, success in achieving family harmony requires quite a lot of give and take, effort, and sincere commitment.

The implications to one's lifestyle as a visually disabled person are similarly profound. How the individual manages living with blindness depends greatly on the outlook one has about life. Living with blindness also depends on managing the completion of daily tasks. Day-to-day needs are not always translated into daily tasks; yet, the individual's wants and needs bear witness to one's outlook on life. It is clear that a positive outlook is extremely important and is something to strive for. Having a positive outlook will help the visually disabled individual find value and meaning in what is a new orientation and approach to life. The fact is that there will be lifestyle changes whether you are a child, young adult, or a mature individual.

The varying degrees of visual impairment pose challenges in determining the lifestyle changes needed. For example, I would have trouble distinguishing one student from another when I worked in the classroom with the lights on. The minute I switched to an activity requiring low vision lighting, my vision would improve dramatically.

When we teachers were notified of upcoming staff meetings, I would obtain the materials for the meeting ahead of time so that I could spend some time reviewing them and making notations in large print of what I wanted to address during the meeting. This gave me a greater ability to participate fully in the discussions taking place. Yet, I confounded my colleagues; they could not fathom how I could participate with the group in a fluid fashion.

These visual acuity nuances also caused mild sensations with my family members. I clearly remember one day when my son was coming to pick me up from work. We had errands to run, and he agreed to meet me at the front entrance. I was there at the appointed time and a car pulled up. I got into the car and greeted my son. The gentleman behind the wheel and I sat staring at each other for a few moments. "Obviously, you are not my son," I said before I quickly exited the car.

Awkward situations are simply part of the inevitable adjustments a disabled individual must make in his or her lifestyle. As a school-teacher, I encountered many such awkward moments. I learned how to face them openly and to find new ways to manage them. I knew I had to learn new skills when I walked the hallways in my school and could not distinguish my friends and colleagues who passed by.

It is frightfully easy to give someone the wrong impression when you are living with a disability. Visual problems in particular create unique emotional reactions in those who are close to us. We are naturally depen-dent on our sense of sight. Our vision helps us stay safe by scanning our environment and screening for dangers within it. It helps us pick things we like and discard what we do not like. Vision is often the first sense engaged when seeking a life partner. Nature nudges us towards healthy individuals who can add positive elements to our genetic line, but our senses, especially our eyes, tell us if we are attracted to that person. It is therefore important to understand how one's visual impairment affects one's daily life.

Living with Cone Rod Dystrophy means that eventually one feels the sadness of not being able to see sharply and in color—not to men-tion the pain caused by sunshine, and the diminished vision one expe-riences in low lighting. The affected individual will forever miss being able to see sunrises, sunsets, the changing colors of the seasons, and the faces of people in his or her life. Perhaps these moments can no longer be experienced exactly as they were lived when one was sighted, but the good news is that they can be enjoyed in new ways. Learning new strategies and skills will open one's to new ways of experiencing impor-tant moments in his or her life. I find that a day at the beach in my native Dominican Republic simply means enduring the sunlight for the pleasure of hearing the waves crashing against the seashore, the cacophony of sounds coming from the birds hovering over the sea, the children playing, and everyone enjoying the day. There is genuine pleasure and thankfulness for being part of the life teeming around me.

When my granddaughter was born, I was still able to focus a bit. My daughter, her husband, and the baby lived with me for two years. Very early on, I was able to forge a bond with my granddaughter that endures today. When she woke up for those infamous two o'clock feedings, I took my turns staying up with her. During these precious moments, I would sing songs and tell her stories. This ritual evolved to the point that when she was a two-year-old, we would wake up early in the morning and have tea and a cookie together. My eyesight continued to grow progressively worse, but our routine never waned. To this day, my granddaughter and I share early morning talks, which she now refers to as "girl talk."

Almost every night I would read *Goodnight Moon* to her. I read that book to her for a long time, and the story would change slightly each night. I could not remember exactly the story line every time. Fortunately, my granddaughter would prompt me when I was not following the story to her satisfaction. The author of that book perhaps never envisioned the twists and turns that my nightly retelling of the story would take, but it was a great pleasure to my granddaughter and me. In fact, as she got older, I often wove into the story whatever had been going on in her day. It really turned out to be a new *Goodnight Moon* story every time. As she got older, she took over the storytelling. The moon eventually had monologues, dialogues, or soliloquies with other characters in the story. My inability to see her face or the writing in the book never interfered with our bonding or enjoyment of these moments. I simply learned to adjust to this new reality. I was able to enjoy all aspects of my life without thinking in terms of limitations. Thankfully, I remember her newborn features, and I was able to see her until she was three years old. She is permanently etched in my memory as a beautiful person for all time.

One of the optical aids that truly helped me to manage the changes in my lifestyle were dark red contact lenses prescribed by my low vision specialist. I'd had to wear dark glasses at all times until I was given these contact lenses. The difference these lenses made on my lifestyle was dramatic. Specifically, I was able to enjoy the outdoors a little more comfortably. The lenses are not designed to improve acuity, however; these lenses filter light so that the individual can feel more comfortable in brightly lit conditions.

So dramatic was the addition of these contacts to my lifestyle that everyone around me noticed. My loved ones, friends, and colleagues noticed how naturally I could move around in the world. I did not have to relegate myself to doing activities only at dusk or at night. When I walked into my school without wearing dark glasses, it caused a sensation. My co-workers were amazed. They remarked repeatedly, "We wondered what you looked like without those glasses." I had gotten so used to wearing dark glasses that I never paid attention to how others felt and reacted to them. Most people like to see into the eyes of others. It is how people generally pick up subtle nuances and changes in facial expressions. The expressions in turn provide clues as to how a person may be feeling, despite what he or she is saying.

Researchers have found that people believe there is deception in someone when that person is unable to look another in the eyes. An individual may even feel threatened by someone who averts his eyes or wears dark glasses. It is not a coincidence that menacing figures or villains in movies, television programs, musical videos, video games, and on the Internet generally wear dark glasses. Conversely, a person may feel more at ease with someone who looks him in the eyes and will go so far as to believe that the person is trustworthy. It is therefore quite understandable when someone feels slightly uneasy around a person wearing dark glasses.

It is especially unsettling when a person wears dark glasses when there is no need to do so. Wearing dark glasses inside a building, at dusk, or at night can cause alarm. Others may feel such a degree of unease that they may actually move away from the wearer of the glasses. In fact, this has happened to me on several occasions, causing me to speculate that there may yet be other reasons why this stir is created. I suspect that one reason, in the case of the visually challenged, is that some people just do not know how to react to a visually disabled person. Reading facial expressions, including gazing into the eyes of another, really does help us determine how best to interact with others using the appropriate behavior for a particular situation.

Today, I am more aware than ever of how others may perceive and react to me as a visually challenged person. This awareness allows me to do whatever I can to put others at ease. As I gain insight about the kind of lifestyle changes I must make, I think about how others react to me; because I value their feelings, I do whatever I can to ease their anxiety. As I go about creating a lifestyle that allows me to be comfortable in the world while living with Cone Rod Dystrophy, these considerations are not only necessary, but ultimately, they are worth the effort.

Each year, due to the progressive nature of my Cone Rod Dystrophy, I lose more of my central acuity. The result is that I can no longer distinguish faces, look at photographs without optical aids, or even watch television. There are as many losses as there are gains. The progression of my Cone Rod Dystrophy has been slow, thereby giving me time to adjust to blindness throughout much of my lifetime. That this progression has been slow has been a blessing. As the changes to my vision occur, I have been able to continue adding to the body of information that I have thus far accumulated in this writing.

As of this moment, I have learned to anticipate when my vision will shift. I will feel light headed for a week or so, and at night, my head will feel heavy. Generally, a week after these symptoms, my eyes will become blurrier. It is then time once again to visit the eye specialist to assure that it is not another type of eye disease; I also visit the low vision specialist for a new assessment on possible optical aids. This is the management of Cone Rod Dystrophy—you stay in control of your life and love living it.

Although I no longer have central acuity, the faces of my loved ones, friends, and colleagues are forever etched in my memory. I remember them just as they were the last time I saw them clearly. To me, that is a gift. Another gain is that my blindness allows me to pay attention to what is important about my interactions with others.

I am blessed to have many special people in my life who love me. I asked one such person some time ago what he thought were the best aspects of our relationship. "Having honest communication, commitment, and time," he said. The same is also true about my personal relationship with my blindness. I strive to be honest with myself about my reality, communicate how I am feeling, discuss my abilities and limitations with those that I love, and make the necessary changes to make sense of my world and enjoy life to the fullest.

When planning for lifestyle changes, reliance on whatever visual ability one has may actually be a secondary concern. A more immediate approach is to learn how to adjust to the loss of vision one is likely to experience. Visual acuity alone is not always a good indicator of the kinds of adjustments you'll need to make in your life. Everyone experiences changes in their vision, especially as they enter the mid-life years. A visually challenged person will experience ongoing and often dramatic changes in visual acuity. These changes can differ from person to person. Someone with good acuity may have difficulties completing certain tasks, while another person with worse acuity will not have any difficulties. A person can use his or her remaining sight to accomplish the tasks that need to be done. Remaining or residual sight can also be enhanced by alternative assistive technologies.

It is important during these lifestyle changes to work with various eye professionals. Low vision specialists, local, state, and federal agencies for the blind and vision impaired, vision rehabilitation services, and other organizations serving this population will provide much help and support to the individual. These resources can offer assistance in determining how much residual visual acuity remains. Vision assessments will establish which alternative optical aids and assistive technologies you can use to enhance your sight. The purpose is to determine your visual needs, determine the degree of vision relative to those needs, and determine which methods are likely to help you pursue your lifestyle activities with enjoyment and success.

One must have a clear understanding of the current demands in one's life when facing the need for lifestyle changes. It is important to be clear about the demands in one's life and the degree of completion necessary to fulfill them in a satisfactory manner. Different situations, tasks, and activities require different levels of energy, commitment, and skill. Logically, this will require different methods for satisfying those demands. Just as all people have differentiated visual needs due to aging, illness, or visual problems, there is no one-size-fits-all method.

Though it can be a time consuming process and often a frustrating one as well, once you learn how your eyes function best and what tools you need, life becomes much easier.

After working closely with your health professionals, the next logical step will be to set achievable goals. This will give you something to strive toward every day. Losing your vision can be so traumatic; without having set goals to achieve, you can easily become engulfed in negativity. For some people, the temptation to give up, and to succumb to the belief that the future is no longer bright, causes them to slide into dependency. I encourage you to resist this temptation and remain strong and positive instead, knowing that you are not alone.

I met a young woman going blind due to retinopathy. She had diabetes and was receiving dialysis. She said that she became more despondent every day. She stopped going out except to receive treatments. She told me that she already felt as if she was dead. Tears came to my eyes as we spoke. This young woman had lost hope and given up on herself. We had a long conversation about faith, motivation, and hope. At the end of the conversation, I felt helpless. I knew I had not spoken the words she needed to hear. I wanted to breathe a little air of hope into her future, just as air is driven into the lungs of a person who has inhaled water. I felt that I had failed.

It is difficult to stay positive under such tough conditions, especially when an individual does not have a caring family, friends, or a support system. Keeping faith and hope alive for the difficult times ahead seems an impossible task. It is essential to reach out to others in one's life. I find it valuable to connect with individuals and groups that are experiencing similar challenges.

This particular strategy works because it is a tried and true mentoring model that attests to the support individuals can give one another. Whether the mentoring takes places within groups such as Alcoholics Anonymous, parent engagement groups in school settings, or even social clubs and social media, this model works very well. It is important to find the professionals, organizations, and groups that can help establish that necessary support system for you.

Setting achievable goals and then meeting them helps you experience immediate reinforcement with every success. Whether these successes are extrinsic or intrinsic, small or phenomenal does not matter. Experiencing them on whatever scale they are achieved is a great motivator.

One of my friends was elated when she learned how to eat without spilling any food. It was a big step for her because her goal was to eat out at her favorite restaurant again. Another friend mastered the tricky art of plugging in an electrical cord so that he could listen to his radio. These may seem like baby steps to some, but for a visually challenged individual, they serve as great motivators to keep learning, doing, and moving forward.

Once achievable goals have been set, an assessment of what you need to fulfill these goals is the next step to take. The assessment should include living strategies, mobility lessons, alternative optical aids, assistive technologies, and other existing tools. The assessment should also encompass a wholistic approach, which includes special attention to the psychosocial, emotional, and physical well-being of the individual. It is just as important to incorporate goals related to nutrition and the role of exercise and vitamin therapy. Again, in this wholistic context, the individual with access to good healthcare is going to reap many benefits. It is essential for visually challenged individuals to have access to affordable healthcare to get the assistance they desperately need from the appropriate health professionals.

Another critical reason for having access to these health professionals is that they assist in the often complicated world of acquiring services from different agencies. They are able to help individuals in acquiring a social security disability designation, transportation services, social services, and reasonable accommodations in the workplace.

One of the earliest decisions you will have to make is in regards to driving privileges. Health professionals can help a visually challenged individual determine whether to continue to drive. Many people associate driving with freedom and independence because driving gives us the freedom to go anywhere we want to go at any time. Implied as well is that one is still capable of mentally and physically handling a car.

Freedom, mental acuity, and physical vigor are fundamental concepts. The underlying message is that if one can drive, then one is "whole." That person still has good reflexes, eyesight, and health. Losing a driver's license due to a health condition, aging, poor eyesight, or any other debilitating condition often equates to being less than whole for some. This may lead a person to feeling valueless. A key element to staying mentally positive is to recognize that the loss of a driver's license does not infringe on one's freedom or independence. It is simply a necessary adjustment to one's lifestyle.

Health professionals will assist in navigating through the myriad issues of concern to the visually challenged. They are versed in deciphering the Americans with Disabilities Act and its implications, which range from managing educational settings and workplace issues to understanding the legislation's impact on activities one does for fun and relaxation.

The roles of low vision specialists, optometrists, ophthalmologists, and other professionals in the field are more than just to help you maximize your functional level of vision. These individuals, as well as the groups, organizations, and agencies they work with, are guides to a new way of living. In particular, support groups for the blind and visually impaired are adept at helping those with reduced visual acuity find the training, tools, and wholistic aid they need. They are trained to help individuals manage their disability, continue enjoying life, and continue moving forward. Rehabilitation professionals—who may or may not be connected to an agency for the blind and visually impaired—can provide advice and training on a variety of areas. They can instruct individuals on how to choose the appropriate low vision lighting and contrast conditions to maximizing one's remaining vision. These professionals also have access to non-visual aids, and can instruct patients in their uses.

How does one continue living and loving life as a blind person? I have to admit that I am still working on loving my blindness because it was an emotional shock to receive the diagnosis. Just as with any other serious illness, once the emotional shock of the disability is accepted, the next step is to bolster oneself and negate any feelings of powerlessness. For each of us, this process is different, and it is not constrained to a particular time frame; only you can decide what support systems you will need. A very good friend always tells me, "You are worthy." There used to be an ad for a hair color where the spokesperson always said the brand name followed by a pause and the phrase, "Because you're worth it." I think this is true in all phases of our lives. We work to overcome our fears, and we seek the things, people, and experiences that will enhance our lives and help us feel happy and productive—and we do this because we are worthy.

Acknowledging our worth, and reveling in our value to our loved ones, community, and society, revives in us the spirit and courage to face our challenges. With renewed courage, we can learn the alternative techniques, strategies, rehabilitations, and other skills needed to be productive. Feeling productive and of value to others and ourselves promotes a desire to have a good quality of life. If we realign and adjust to the disability we have, happiness can be in our future. Living and loving life as a blind person is absolutely possible.

Researchers in psychosomatic medicine have found that many patients who lose all of their vision actually feel better emotionally because they have learned the necessary rehabilitative techniques they need for a good quality of life. I can relate to this. When I think back on the times I had to go for an annual vision exam and have my eyes dilated, I remember the panic and anxiety I suffered every time and how overwhelming and debilitating it was. Dilating my eyes incapacitated my vision to the point of blindness. During those moments, I felt it would be better to be totally blind. I asked one of my friends from the National Federation for the Blind whether it bothered him to have his eyes dilated. He said, "Not anymore!" When you can accept the fact that you will possibly become totally blind, and you learn alternative techniques to live daily life successfully, then the prospect of whatever will happen to your vision no longer makes you scared, anxious, and panic-stricken. You regain control over yourself and your situation.

When you accept your condition and its ultimate outcome, it is easier to motivate yourself to learn new skills and thus attain a happier, more stable life. I have finally accepted and embraced my ongoing blindness. I am learning to live with new lifestyle changes. Most importantly, I am learning to love myself all over again as a blind person. In the end, this is the greater goal—to continue loving life as a blind individual.

CHAPTER 6:
SOUNDS OF JOY

*Practical concerns for managing daily tasks,
working, and living a full life*

Exploring the very nature of what it is to be blind has been a consuming passion of mine. Reading literature on the subject has been instrumental in this understanding. Likewise, I have gained so much value in reading about the lives and experiences of others such as Louis Braille, Ray Charles, Stevie Wonder, and Helen Keller, and simply by talking with friends in my support groups. Just as important in this understanding is the feedback I receive from others as to how they perceive me.

A great part of my new reality is accepting that I can be a troubling element to others. To some, I may be an actual annoyance or inconvenience. Blind and visually challenged individuals can enlighten others and help them understand what it's like by engaging in open, honest communication about their condition with those around them, and by honestly sharing how others can facilitate their movements through their daily activities. Being knowledgeable about your eye condition and being able to articulate and impart this knowledge often places others at ease and gives them the green light to ask questions and learn more from the most likely source—you. It is also likely that when the individual who is visually challenged is skilled at completing daily tasks, job responsibilities, and managing relationships, she bolsters her own confidence while impressing this on others. Being skilled and confident are valued concepts in every society.

As a sighted person, I learned the tools and skills I needed to overcome the challenges I would find in society and in particular, the workplace. As a Latino young person, and specifically a poor immigrant from the Dominican Republic, the negative perceptions of others or their misplaced pity and charity were all barriers that I had to overcome.

Many communities within the American society of the early 1970s were undergoing similar experiences. This was particularly the case for ethnic and cultural groups in places like Englewood, New Jersey, where an islander was seen through the same racial, cultural, and ethnic prisms as other minority cultural groups were. When I was coming of age, my understanding of these paradigms grew. My energies and efforts were focused on getting the best education possible. I realized that to progress and prosper in American society, there was no time to waste; an education was paramount to achieving these ends. There was an even greater reason for my desire to be educated. The reason was due to the messages I heard from the church we attended. Groups that served the underprivileged, such as the Urban League and Upward Bound, and caring teachers all told us to learn everything we could to become knowledgeable in an area of expertise, to gain academic skills, and to earn a degree. This helped us feel better about ourselves and gave us the competence and confidence to prosper. Further, the message implied was that others would now see us in a different light.

Having achieved the goal of graduating from high school, going to college posed the next great difficulty. Challenges abounded on a daily basis, from concerns about how to pay for a college education to managing freedom and responsibility, and making good decisions as to living in a dormitory while maintaining good grades. I was determined to prove that I could compete at a university and be successful. Indeed, I did excel, and I went on to establish a career as a classroom teacher.

As a sighted individual, the person that I knew myself to be was someone who faced realities, concerns, and challenges in life head on. I always expected to have positive outcomes if I did my part and worked hard at whatever I needed to accomplish. When I was finally diagnosed with Cone Rod Dystrophy, which meant I knew that visual impairment and blindness would be in my future, I did not cease to be myself. Yet, there were subtle changes in my behavior and in my mind that told me how deeply the diagnosis had affected me.

Gradually, I became less certain of myself and less sure of where I was going and what I was supposed to be doing. Ironically, this increased the more I learned about my eye condition. I was afraid of my future. I worried about how I would take care of my children and myself. Very subtly, I noted that my colleagues at work and others around me did not know how to approach me, what to say, and (horrors) what *not* to say to me.

Some people offered condolences, as if I had a terminal illness and was going to die. Others became overly solicitous of me. They wanted to literally pick me up in their arms and take me wherever I had to go or do for me whatever I needed to do. Yet, others insisted through their reactions that they were going to treat me like a "normal" person—no coddling and no excuses. Curiously, very few people in my life actually wanted to talk about my eye condition or to know what the experience of blindness was like for me. So rare was it to have someone inquire about my experiences that I was surprised when a very good friend asked me to describe what being visually impaired was like for me. One day, out of curiosity, I asked him why he wanted to know. He simply said, "I want to understand."

There they were—the very words that helped me realize that I had not done my part. It is sometimes easy to place the blame on everyone around us. Some of us who are disabled wait for others to approach us first as if it is their fault that no contact has been made between us. In talking to other disabled friends, I know that at times we feel we are "sparing" others from having to interact with us in order to avoid an awkward conversation. In neither situation are we offering understanding. There seems to be a dichotomy in what people feel and expect about the blind and visually challenged. Perhaps this mirrors the very same ambivalence we feel. These reactions are common. Society includes numerous unfortunate examples of how we are leery of talking to each other about difficult yet meaningful things. Look no further than our public discourse surrounding issues affecting, the minorities, the gay, the poor, the rich, and the troubled—but especially, the different.

Given these varying views in societal structures such as our workplace, relationships, and the number of social activities we engage in on a daily basis, blind and visually challenged individuals must be open to fostering honest and truthful interactions. We begin the process of understanding when we share the truth about our condition and how it affects the people around us. As we proceed toward a future of living happy and productive lives, we will need others to understand what that journey is all about and offer assistance along the way.

CHAPTER 7:
TALKING TO OTHERS ABOUT CONE ROD DYSTROPHY

Learning to love oneself as a blind or visually challenged person and coping with emotional issues and stages of sadness and loss while helping family, friends, and others adapt to new realities

One of the things that characterizes the nature of human beings is the complexity and dynamism in our interactions and relationships with one another. Whether sighted or not, we all have the need and capacity to make significant emotional connections with others. We don't always follow through on developing the potential that this drive inspires. Some of us fall short for a variety of reasons; perhaps when we experience emotional turmoil, loneliness, and even alienation. For others, it takes supreme effort not to succumb to these negative aspects and forge ahead, determined to relate to others, establish meaningful relationships, and find happiness.

Recently, a very good friend died. He passed away in the night alone. He was not found until the following morning. It struck me that we do not have a choice as to how we are born or who is in the room to greet us into the world. Most of us do have this choice by the time we are facing this finite moment in our mortal transition. It may be that the mark of a happy and well-lived life, or at least our attempt at it, lies in how we transition at this ultimate moment and who is there to help us through it. Most of us are therefore part of a chain of complex and confounding relationships. We are individuals with our own particular propensities, but we are also daughters, sons, brothers, sisters, aunts, uncles, husbands, wives, girlfriends, boyfriends, partners, mothers, fathers, grandmothers, and grandfathers.

Quite clearly, some relationships work well—others, not so much. Most of the time, we use all of our senses to gather information about each other during interactions together. Regardless of whether the relationship is a personal or professional one, or even a passing acquaintance, we look at someone's facial expressions and body language, in addition to their words, to determine how we are going to react. Following verbal and visual cues can be challenging but necessary if we want to establish meaningful, healthy relationships in our lives. A visually challenged person does not have the entire range of sensory cues that sighted people have; therefore, visually challenged individuals, by necessity, must rely on senses other than vision to aid them in their human interactions.

In the case of the blind and visually impaired individual, the other senses may be affected as well. Quite often, with visual impairments and total blindness, there may be some additional disabilities. Where Cone Rod Dystrophy is concerned, as vision continues to degenerate, the individual's hearing may also becomes less reliable. Cone Rod Dystrophy patients often also experience changes to their equilibrium. Of course, it must be noted that some of these changes may also be due to aging. In spite of these possible effects, the sense of hearing, touch, smell, and locomotion are very important to the visually challenged individual.

When a visually impaired individual is unable to see someone's face or read that person's body language, and must rely on cues afforded through other senses, he or she becomes more attuned to smells, body positioning, nuances in the voice, and other messages relayed through touch and proximity. Visualization is another skill that may be developed. This is the capacity to see where an object is located, where a person is situated, or what his or her face or body are expressing by using the remaining senses. To understand what this might be like, the next time you are on the phone with someone, pay attention to the nuances in the person's voice. Is what he or she saying in sync with the way it is being said? That is, what are his or her tone, intonation, rhythm, and word patterns suggesting? Do you get the feeling that much has been said without any real meaning, or has a world of significance been imparted to you with a minimum of words? These are the tools and skills that the visually impaired and blind person will have to fine-tune in order to develop dynamic, positive, and intimate working relationships. Those who are blind and visually impaired become adept, with practice, to these subtle changes.

The motivation for learning and using these skills is the same for us all. Most of us need to feel close to others, to foster good relationships, and to fall in love. When we learn these skills as visually impaired and blind individuals, we may share them with others. Simple exercises, such as the telephone exercise cited above, can help the people in our lives understand our reality. Many support groups, local organizations, and state government/federally-sponsored programs for the blind and vision impaired offer information, classes, and other forms of help to the families and friends of the individual with a visual challenge. Engaging in these activities will help others relate in a more productive fashion with the visually challenged individual.

My family members are familiar with how I use a cane, and are comfortable walking along with me, listening for oncoming traffic, and being aware of a number of realities I encounter when outdoors. They have learned to describe our experiences so that I can participate fully. Describing locales, colors, shifting seasons, and the sights they see as we travel along helps me offer appropriate and thoughtful comments. It is important to be aware of and demand your place in the family structure. Just because you are blind or visually impaired does not mean you have lost your mind. You can still offer your children advice and guidance, you can be supportive in your loving relationships, and you can still be a devoted son or daughter. Indoors, my family has adjusted to my need for low vision lighting and the labeling of clothing, appliances, and entryways. We have realized that minimizing the spaces where I need to walk helps me avoid purple shins and overturned furniture.

Everyone will be happier when the entire family can adapt to the challenges facing the visually impaired or blind individual. No matter how much or how little they can relate to the individual's experiences, this will benefit everyone. The primary benefit, of course, is to help them become familiar, comfortable, or even skilled with the tools that the visually challenged family member must use. Many of those around you who are involved in your life will welcome learning, growing, and following your lead. One is simply giving them the confidence to feel comfortable with you, your disability, and the accommodations that are needed for you to continue having healthy relationships. Those who are around you will look to you for guidance in how to behave in a way that is comfortable for them and for you. If you are shaken, uncertain, afraid, and not able to evolve, there is little motivation for them to do so. Some principles that we strive to live by are difficult to achieve. People often say practice makes perfect, and this is quite true.

First, it is important for you to learn everything about your condition so that you can educate your friends and family members. Become knowledgeable about what it is and what the treatment options are. Encourage questioning within yourself and in others. Let them become involved in the care and management of your condition to whatever degree is necessary. I have found great joy in knowing that those around me have cared to learn about my condition. They want to understand the skills I need in order to function, and they try to learn them as well. They have been helpful simply by being mindful of the accommodations that I require in diverse settings. I can dine out, travel, go to the movies, the theatre, or any venue with my family and friends and enjoy the outing as much as they do. For those who do not have a family support system, groups and organizations abound that can be helpful in this regard. You never need to be alone in managing your visual challenges.

Second, I now know that it is just as important to practice being brave. Face the future as courageously as you can. I have been fortunate in that my condition allows me to adjust gradually as my vision diminishes. I have been able to prepare for the next stage of vision loss. Yet, even so, fear of the unknown is always present. Knowledge can minimize fear. Sharing your fears with loved ones, doctors, support groups, or others in your life can help to overcome many of the fears. I tell myself *Don't be afraid*, over and over, and I become a warrior on behalf of my own cause.

Third, be committed to learning the skills needed to live productively. The visually challenged person can learn to be as independent as possible. From learning how to sew a button with the right tools to eating a meal at a restaurant, learning new things brings new challenges and excitement.

Finally, it is rewarding to discover inner strength that you did not know was there. Summarily, the blind or visually impaired person has to be committed to learning all there is to know about her eye condition, and she needs to keep up with new information on the subject. The visually impaired or blind individual can definitely continue to live a happy and productive life doing most if not all the activities she has always done; all she needs is a repertoire of effective living and managing skills.

These are valuable skills in everyday living, but perhaps most importantly, they are marketable skills that allow the visually impaired person to continue being productive in the workplace. The knowledge and skills acquired can be shared with others to help them become part of your experience. Sharing your experience with others is another form of learning about yourself. All of these activities simply point to the fact that you value and are devoted to your personal growth and that you care for other people, and they in turn are a testament to your ability to face the future as courageously as possible.

Loving yourself as a visually impaired or blind person is as much a process as it is a state of being. It is a process of devotion to yourself and your development in your journey toward self-actualization. Everyone has a need to be happy and productive. The blind and visually impaired are no different. A person who is challenged with any limiting condition does not lose his humanity. Just like anyone else, when you open yourself to new experiences and you are committed to learning new things, very positive outcomes will surely follow. I am learning to embrace my blindness, and I expect bright days always ahead.

CHAPTER 8:
CURRENT EYE RESEARCH TRENDS

*What studies reveal about Cone Rod Dystrophy
and the future of research on eye conditions*

Many researchers studying Cone Rod Dystrophy have determined that no cure currently exists. The treatment options available are, as of this writing, severely limited and unreliable. In fact, there are no treatments beyond the use of alternative optical implements such as dark lenses. Cone Rod Dystrophy patients are advised to use dark glasses to protect their retinas from bright lights.

However, there is good news for the future. Researchers working in the field of gene research seem to have identified genes that may be involved in the condition. This is exciting because it means that eventually, this work will lead to answers that now escape us. Gene research can answer how and why the condition presents itself, as well as who may be at risk and where and when it occurs.

Discovery of genes related to this condition will lead to gene therapies that may offer a cure one day. Imagine a day when retinal diseases such as Cone Rod Dystrophy or Retinitis Pigmentosa can be cured through gene replacement therapy or some other means of manipulation resulting from these exciting studies. The future may be closer than we can dream.

Although it is difficult to cite the most current treatment for Cone Rod Dystrophy, we can keep up with current research. Contacting the most well-known centers engaged in research activity for Cone Rod Dystrophy is as easy as talking to your eye specialist, joining a support group, contacting state or federal agencies or organizations involved in this area, or searching the Internet. To aid in this search, here are some of the most well-known centers in the United States.

The National Institutes for Health (NIH)

The Kellogg Eye Center

Johns Hopkins University

The Georgetown Center for Sight

The Foundation Fighting Blindness

Living with Cone Rod Dystrophy means keeping abreast of current information available while also managing one's life effectively. Learning to manage your life as a Cone Rod Dystrophy patient allows you to live independently, move around your environment safely, interact appropriately with others, manage daily tasks with confidence, and continue working and contributing to your community and society. Living with Cone Rod Dystrophy ultimately means loving yourself as a valued, capable, and worthy visually impaired or blind individual.

CHAPTER 9:
PARENTS OF CHILDREN WITH CONE ROD DYSTROPHY

Staying positive and teaching children necessary skills and coping mechanisms

As a child growing up in the Dominican Republic, no one within my family was aware of my eye condition. Although there were many visual issues among the women in my family, they were generally attributed to old age, malnutrition, injury, or the lack of adequate health care. In fact, the only manifestation of my visual impairment was an aversion to bright light. Being light sensitive while growing up on an island is not something that concerned anyone—it is to be expected. My family never considered that my sensitivity to light was a signal for more serious visual problems.

Provided there is a concern, and the family takes very seriously the complaints voiced by children in such cases, much can be done to slow the effects of many visual conditions. Even in the best-case scenarios where children do have access to good health care, parents of children with Cone Rod Dystrophy often feel uncertain and inadequate regarding what to do. This is the case with many retinal conditions, as there are still no cures; parents experience many conflicted feelings. In addition to feeling uncertain about what to do for their child, as was the case with my parents, they may also feel helpless, hopeless, anxious, and even guilty.

Before these feelings become overwhelming, it is important for parents to gain a full understanding of what the condition is and how it will affect the child as he or she grows older. In this way, the parent is best equipped to help the child. Some parents may need to seek counseling for themselves and others in the family to deal with the emotional distress they feel. It is normal for parents to feel that they have passed on a genetic flaw to their child. Mothers may feel that they did something during pregnancy to cause the condition.

Learning about the condition—its heredity or its physiological gene aberration that might be particular to the individual—may help in alleviating these feelings of guilt. It is also quite natural for parents to feel less than positive about their child's future. Parents worry about everything from the time their child is born through his or her adult years. The knowledge that the eye condition will lead to visual impairment or total blindness is terrifying to most parents facing this situation. Staying positive is necessary in order to feel hopeful and to help the child learn how to live a happy and productive life with the condition.

It is all right to feel bad about what is happening to one's child. It is not all right to be so overwhelmed with grief and feelings of guilt for "giving" the child the condition that one becomes unable to cope and therefore unable to help the child learn coping mechanisms. A healthy understanding of genes and chromosomes can help parents feel better. Not only will they know how to deal with the effects of the condition, they will also know what their child might contribute to his or her future children. Ultimately, the overriding reason for staying positive and being hopeful is to allow the visually impaired or blind child to continue to grow in a healthy and happy way. The point is that a child is still a child who just happens to have vision loss due to a visual disorder such as Cone Rod Dystrophy. Of course, children will want to do all the things that other children do. Parents, by necessity, will need to know when to let them actively participate in everyday activities and when safety is an issue that forces them to curtail or redirect some of those activities. In the early days of the child's development, parents will often need to gently intervene due to their child's limitations that may be present. As the child learns the skills needed to stay safe when participating in most activities, these interventions may lessen.

Parents will help their children by accepting the reality of their child's visual impairment or blindness, gaining knowledge of the condition, staying positive, and by teaching their children the necessary skills and coping mechanisms he or she will need in order to deal with the condition. In this way, the parents will experience a more positive outlook and diminish negative feelings while ensuring that their child will live a happier and more productive life.

As children with Cone Rod Dystrophy develop, families will have much assistance from a diverse group of professionals, organizations, and agencies. Parents will receive the first of such assistance from pediatricians and other medical staff attending their child. These professionals will likely uncover, perhaps through regular exams and parental input, the ways in which the child's eyes are functioning. As time goes on, eye professionals will increasingly become more important in the life of the family by more extensive tests, which may lead to a diagnosis. In addition, during the school years, teachers, counselors, and other school support personnel will also become very important to the family whose child has Cone Rod Dystrophy. Establishing good relationships among the school staff involved with the child is the best way to meet the child's needs.

Most importantly, open and honest communication between the parent and school personnel is the key to a happy school life for children with Cone Rod Dystrophy. This type of communication among the people involved with the child guarantees that school-age children with this visual impairment will have the assistive technology, academic assistance, and emotional support they need. In a collaborative effort, the school will help the family by providing children with specialized programs, learning accommodations, and learning tools to ensure the child's academic success. Just as importantly, parents must insist that the school personnel see the child's eye condition in a positive light. Just as parents must stay positive and look toward the future with hope, so must the school staff. Staying positive and helping children cope and manage their vision loss is good for the parent, the child, and the school.

As children with Cone Rod Dystrophy transition to the teen years, along with ongoing, normal teen concerns with school, there may be a host of new issues related to the visual condition. They may feel different because of their situation. Although not as prevalent today as in previous decades, concerns regarding how other children view those that are involved in individualized education programs remain. There have been cases where children have experienced low self-esteem and a negative self-image because they were in special education. These perceptions have been reinforced in schools where these programs are under appreciated. The school must set a more positive tone, from the principal to the building management crews. Children who are involved in individualized education programs must be allowed to integrate fully into school life; this will mitigate feelings of alienation. In addition to providing the necessary tools to ensure academic success, the school environment can be supportive of the emotional, social, and psychological growth of the visually impaired or blind child.

Along with the cited concerns above, new vision-related issues could surface during the school years. Some children with Cone Rod Dystrophy may notice a change in the way they see colors along with blurred vision and sensitivity to light. In fact, some children may no longer be able to discern colors correctly, or will see them in duller hues. They may mistake one color for another. Since Cone Rod Dystrophy can affect individuals in different ways, others may retain their ability to see colors from only one particular part of the spectrum. Yet for others, they will experience, over time, a loss of color recognition altogether.

A normal part of the teen years is the desire to be social—going out with friends to the movies and other social activities. Meeting other young people and dating consumes much of the teen's attention. In particular, learning to drive and finally being able to drive solo has become a marker for maturing, being grown up, and gaining independence. Teens with Cone Rod Dystrophy may notice difficulty when shopping with friends by being unable to distinguish colors. They may have trouble watching movies at the movie theatre, and driving may become a safety issue. As the challenges surface and cause concern within the teen, he or she may feel uncomfortable in social situations and perhaps begin to withdraw from friends and family, and avoid once-favorite activities.

Parents who have developed open and honest lines of communication with their teen will be alert to these changes. More than ever, the teen with Cone Rod Dystrophy needs to know what these changes are, how they affect them, and what strategies and skills they will need to adjust to and manage these changes. Parents will need to convey over and over again that the teen is not alone in this struggle. The school should also be there to support them. In no way should teens with Cone Rod Dystrophy envision a bleak future in which they cannot cope with the changes in their vision. Many Cone Rod Dystrophy patients have gradual changes in vision. Thus, the teen has time to adjust to the vision loss and learn the necessary skills for independent living.

Continuing to exhibit a positive attitude with teens will help them overcome these feelings and face challenges logically and systematically. Recognizing limitations and managing vision loss will help teens feel in control, and will help them understand their strengths and weaknesses. Involving teens in the planning of activities, in learning more about their condition, and sorting out what they can expect to go through as time goes on is a healthy way for them to manage vision loss and live a full and happy life.

Keeping a journal is a very good way of tracking the progress of the eye condition. Journal writing will also help teens discuss their feelings and experiences as their vision loss progresses. Teens may choose to share the journal with their eye doctors, family, and friends or they may not. For some people, the journal writings are personal and intimate—a bearing of their inner selves that they may not want to share. It becomes an outlet for their innermost feelings. Journal writing can provide eye professionals with a great deal of information regarding the different stages in the teen's vision loss. A journal is also something that parents and other family members can keep. The writing can be used as a comparison of different perspectives on the affected person's loss of vision. Siblings can talk about what they observe in their brother or sister and how it makes them feel. Parents may assuage some of what they are feeling by encouraging them to keep a journal as well. Fathers and mothers can exchange their journals to compare what they are both observing. In the final analysis, all of the efforts that the family and others engage in remind the young person that blindness is a state of being, just as being a teenager is.

Many Cone Rod Dystrophy patients are diagnosed in their early adult years when they are transitioning to the workplace or college. A young adult who has planned her life and has already embarked on what she will be doing for a large part of her life will feel as if destiny has dealt her a fatal blow with a diagnosis of Cone Rod Dystrophy. Some may feel overwhelmed, angry, and even despondent, as their plans seem to have been jeopardized by the diagnosis. Unfortunately, some may even feel hopelessness. For these individuals, seeing a counselor is advisable in order to deal with the emotional impact of being told one is going blind. If this is happening to you, it may be difficult to begin this process, but doing so will help you regain a sense that a good quality of life is still possible. Life can and must move forward as you continue engaging in normal activities. The management of vision loss truly begins with a positive attitude. It can be a long road toward regaining that positive attitude if you feel overwhelmed with despair, but it is important to find the courage to begin the journey.

As the young adult contemplates whether to pursue a job or continue undergraduate education, a good deal of information will be required. If the plan is to join the workforce, working through a job counselor or through local state or federal rehabilitation services is a good place to start. In this setting, the individual learns about the various jobs available to the disabled. He or she can also learn about the Americans with Disabilities Act and how it is implemented in the workplace. Workshops, seminars, and coaching sessions will be offered to help the individual transition quickly into the job market. Whether the person wants to work in the private or public sector, or in federal, state, or county government, the opportunities are there and the limits are only those that the individual imposes on himself.

For those who decide to continue with their education, colleges, universities, institutes, and other centers of learning also provide the assistance visually impaired students need to excel. It is important to understand that by law, academic settings are required to help students with disabilities, and they are equipped to do so. Just as for the school age child, communicating the needs of the college student and providing a framework for how the student will manage academic life is important. Once again, parents are encouraged to help their child when needed, and to know when to allow him or her to experience life independently. Just as with any young adult experiencing total independence for the first time, there will be moments when it is appropriate for parents to intervene.

When I was diagnosed with Cone Rod Dystrophy, I had completed my master's degree and was planning to continue my education and seek a doctorate. After receiving the diagnosis, I began to feel as if I had to change my life plan. I was convinced that I had to let go of my dream of obtaining a doctorate in order to deal with the eye condition. Each of my days, from morning to night, was focused on the fear of going blind. These thoughts became central to my being and displaced all other thoughts. It was a struggle just to get through the day and fulfill my responsibilities to my family and career. Cone Rod Dystrophy issues had taken over. Rather than integrate it into my life activities and manage the effects of the condition, I allowed Cone Rod Dystrophy to become my singular focus and obsession. Every vision change caused me anguish. Every anguished thought fed my obsession. It seemed as though my lifelong dreams were being jeopardized. They seemed to be more illusion than reality. I blamed it all on my cursed fate. In fact, Cone Rod Dystrophy was not changing my life; I was changing my direction, and that direction was down. At the time, I was also experiencing turmoil in my personal life. It all seemed physically overwhelming and emotionally debilitating. It was all I could do to get up every morning and move through the day with some sense of purpose.

As I often did during these years, I went home to the Dominican Republic seeking a little peace for my anguished mind. During my most troubled times, I would always go back and find comfort there. I spent many days in communion with my family, friends, and going to church, and these activities were a godsend. I also spent countless hours walking along the beach at dusk searching for an answer as I looked out over the vast and limitless expanse of the Caribbean Sea. Thinking of the support my family had always given me had a healing effect. It seemed that in a moment of clarity, I reaffirmed what I had always known. If I did not step up to face my challenges, I would have no one to blame for sinking like a stone in the deepest reaches of the sea. There would be no one to rescue me. I came back home to the United States with renewed faith and confidence and started the journey toward self-discovery.

My journey continues today, and it has allowed me to discover my strengths and bolster my weaknesses. Ten years after my epiphany on the beach, I pursued a doctorate in human services. I found that colleges are very adept at helping visually disabled students adjust to the rigors of study. The key is to overcome one's fear and reach out for assistance. In my institution of learning, a program had been designed to aid disabled students achieve academic success. I was assigned a counselor who worked with me in developing my course of study by directing me to the necessary accommodations and resources available on and off campus. These counselors also communicated effectively with my professors to clarify the effects of my visual impairment and to help them understand how Cone Rod Dystrophy would affect my academic work. In addition, these counselors also helped me obtain financial aid.

There are many outside resources that institutions of learning may link to in order to help disabled students. One source made available to me was Recordings for the Blind and Dyslexic (RFBD), a service that provides audio textbooks for the visually disabled student. Through the college, I was able to purchase helpful assistive technologies at a discount, such as a Victor Reader. These and many other accommodations were offered to me as an off-campus student. Those who are on-campus residents have even more accommodations, including accessibility in all buildings and venues.

As I have mentioned, students want to feel independent and in control during their college years. Yet, parents are still a comforting presence and are able to intervene if necessary. Certainly, it is important for students to communicate clearly, honestly, and frequently with their professors. As stated, college counselors will do quite a lot to aid in this process. Success is achievable. To be successful, the communication between doctors, campus offices, professors, and other staff is essential.

Adults diagnosed with a disability while still working may feel as if they will no longer be productive on the job. The opposite is very often the case. Adults with disabilities who are still in the workplace may be even more productive. Disabled workers are not only skilled in the jobs they are trained to do, but they can also acquire new skills to manage their disability. Disabled workers are good workers and should be of value in the workplace because they are greatly motivated to continue working at a high level of productivity. When the employer establishes a support system that works with the disabled worker and develops diversity training with a focus on disability issues, everyone benefits, particularly supervisors. This kind of support and training can often be incorporated into existing training programs with little cost to the employer. Employers may also have assistance from local, state, and federal entities in accommodating the needs of a disabled worker.

Individuals with Cone Rod Dystrophy are likely to continue to do their job successfully. The workplace will retain a valued worker and preserve his/her dignity with honest understanding of the employer, system support and training for other staff members to understand disabled workers, clear objectives addressing accommodation issues, appropriate assistive technologies, and the desire of the worker to do his or her very best.

I thought I had to give up my career as a classroom teacher because I was going blind. Some employers, rather than discourage this feeling in their valued workers consciously or subconsciously, encourage this train of thought. It may be a case of the employer covertly or overtly encouraging an older and more expensive worker to retire, and thereby saving the employer money. At other times, the insensitivity of the staff acts as a discouraging factor. It is incumbent upon the disabled employee to find out what his rights are through a study of the Americans with Disabilities Act (ADA). The worker should also involve his doctor in this process.

The doctor can verify and explain the disabling condition to the employer, and detail how the condition will affect the individual's work. Additionally, doctors and other professionals will consult with the employer regarding proper accommodations and assistive technologies. Even with a high level of communication, a disabled worker must stay vigilant in order to safeguard her position. Some employers might notice a marked change in the disabled employee's demeanor as the disability progresses, even as they comply with regulations of the Americans with Disabilities Act.

The decision to retire or resign from a position should be the disabled worker's decision only. Disabled workers should be able to stay in the workplace for as long as other workers are able to stay if they are given the appropriate tools and a measure of stability in their condition and productivity. Even with workers who have progressive conditions, the accommodations process should be fluid and subject to adjustment as the condition progresses. In fact, it is a viable action for some workers with progressive conditions to retrain for a field that is more compatible with their disability. Training programs designed for the disabled are available through community sources. Rather than regretting forced choices, the disabled worker must do her part by seeking information that will help her fulfill her life plan. I decided to retrain myself in the field of social service, and eventually, I was able to re-enter the workforce. Working adults who have been diagnosed with a disability should not be pressured to retire early, nor should they be forced out of their jobs by their employers. Knowing one's rights under the ADA is the first priority.

The day has hopefully come when disabled workers are sought, recruited, and hired for the valuable workers they are. Along with the human resources personnel policy booklet, workers should be given the ADA booklet; the should also be informed of the employer's program or process for assisting individuals with disabilities and given access to diversity training opportunities for all staff members. As the workforce in the United States ages, more individuals will potentially experience a disability of some kind. The humanity of the workplace is to look beyond the "bottom line" to the asset that a disabled worker can be for an organization. A seasoned, experienced disabled worker can offer years of continued productivity, while a newly hired disabled worker brings unique creativity to the workplace.

Individuals with Cone Rod Dystrophy can look forward to living full, happy, and productive lives while managing the condition. However, this requires a clear understanding of the condition, a willingness to learn new skills and strategies, and to learn how to use appropriate adaptive technologies. Creating links with organizations, centers, and local, state, and federal agencies designed to help the disabled will give access to needed information, resources, equipment, and emotional support. Above all, it is important to develop and keep a positive attitude that includes seeking counseling or support groups if necessary. A positive attitude will likely yield more positive outcomes, which in turn can promote high self-esteem. These elements are the basic building blocks toward maintaining an overall healthy body, mind, spirit, and lifestyle.

CHAPTER 10:
HEALTHY LIVING MATTERS

Focus on a regimen to include nutrition, exercise,
and preventative care

When it comes to keeping your eyes healthy, your physical and mental health play a role, too. Any discussion on maintaining good health will focus on nutrition, exercise, positive lifestyle changes, and wellness of mind and spirit. It is abundantly clear, given research and studies undertaken over the last few decades, that good nutrition can combat many illnesses. The current debate on childhood obesity, sparked by First Lady Michelle Obama, shines a spotlight on the need to encourage healthy eating and exercise for everyone. Much of the research seems to indicate that eating good foods, exercising, initiating positive lifestyle changes, and focusing on the wellness of mind and spirit can be healing for all kinds of health conditions. Given the preponderance of recorded evidence on this subject, one can deduce that in many instances, a sound, healthy body will lead to a reduction or eradication of many illnesses.

In this basic argument, it is fair to assume that a healthy body affects all parts of the body in positive ways, including the eyes. Healthy bodies promote healthy eyes. Obviously, there are eye conditions that stem from genetic flaws or mutations. In addition to genetic and individual predispositions, there are also eye disorders, illnesses, injuries, and other circumstances that are capable of causing irreparable damage to the eyes. Yet, setting all of these considerations aside for the moment, there is great benefit in focusing on nutrition, exercise, and positive lifestyle changes in the area of eye health. This benefit is applied whether an individual has severe eye impairment or not. A friend of mine who was diagnosed with Retinitis Pigmentosa (RP) recently shared with me that she also has Cone Rod Dystrophy. I was surprised and somewhat alarmed. It must have shown in my face because she quickly assured me, "Other than that, I am in perfect condition."

Establishing a regimen to include good nutrition and exercise has become a challenge for people around the world, and particularly in the United States. Sedentary lifestyles, poor eating habits, and the effects of stress have all combined to create a population of unhealthy people. To begin a healthy regimen, it is advisable to develop a plan with the help of a doctor and other health professionals. Optimally, the plan will be based on values and rules that an individual can live by and integrate into a daily routine. It is clear that this is a difficult challenge; hence, the overwhelming numbers of people who are obese and suffering from illnesses associated with obesity.

A logical first step may be to examine the influences, values, habits, and beliefs that operate in one's life, and whether those are positive or negative factors. One only has to note the different attitudes of individuals in our society whose habits promote wellness or a deterioration of their health. It is a known fact that positive influences in life promote overall wellness. Conversely, negative influences affect our lives in negative ways. A good healthy regimen developed in conjunction with a doctor, nutritionist, physical trainer, and other health professionals maximizes the positive, healthy habits and minimizes the negative ones. Maximizing good healthy habits and minimizing unhealthy ones is in everyone's best interest.

The prescriptions for keeping body, mind, and spirit healthy will do the same for the eyes. Not only does a healthy regimen make a positive impact on diseases such as diabetes, high blood pressure/hypertension, and other health problems, but it also keeps the eyes healthy.

For most people, keeping their eyes healthy is a matter of good nutrition, exercise, and positive lifestyle changes. The focus on lifestyle changes is important since these make a difference in our ability to deal effectively with daily stressors. In particular, paying attention to our minds and spirits is optimal in aiding the healing of our bodies. One of the areas of study among those who suffer from Post Traumatic Stress Disorder is the extent to which successfully addressing the mental issues promotes a more rapid healing of the body. The studies being done suggest that attention has to be given to both the mind and body simultaneously. The healing of the mind and the spirit go hand in hand with the healing of the body.

Persons with visual impairments may not have optimal use of their vision, but they can diminish the possibility of acquiring additional eye diseases through routine visual exams and a healthy regimen. Having vision loss does not sanction neglect in keeping one's body healthy. Good nutrition, exercise, and control of harmful diseases are all good for maintaining healthy vision .

When I was diagnosed with Cone Rod Dystrophy, I took note of my overall health condition. As a young person and throughout my child-bearing years, I practiced fairly good health routines. Especially during the child-bearing years, women with good access to healthcare, with the help of health professionals and through routine examinations, should maintain good health. I consumed healthy foods, exercised daily, omitted negative factors, such as exposure to cigarette smoke and other toxins, and meditated each day to de-stress. As I got older and concentrated on other things such as my career, taking care of my family, and running my household, this healthy regimen became less important to me. My healthy regimen disappeared entirely by the time I reached midlife.

For some people, a sudden and serious illness, such as a heart attack, stroke, or diagnosis of diabetes, awakens them to the fact that they have to make changes to their lifestyle. President Bill Clinton remarked in a widely televised interview on health that his heart attack made him change his eating habits. Yet other people may simply note that their body has changed somehow and not for the better. They are motivated to get specific screenings to determine if there is a problem. The diagnosis of Cone Rod Dystrophy was my wake-up call. Although I understood that this eye condition was rooted in genetic factors, in my mind, unhealthy living exacerbated it. I was determined to reassess my eating habits, exercise modes or lack thereof, and my overall lifestyle. My first step was to establish a set of rules to live by that would reflect the healthy routine.

In consultation with a nutritionist, I developed some rules for healthy living: good eating habits (I found that juicing is very energizing), exercising at least twenty minutes each day, and placing a renewed emphasis on activities to help me reduce stress. In fact, engaging in exercise is a great way to lessen stress. Simply walking, swimming, or working with hand weights at a safe pace works wonders.

CHAPTER 11:
RULES TO LIVE BY FOR HEALTHY LIFESTYLES

Developing a set of rules based on your value system
for a healthy body and healthy eyes

Developing a set of healthy rules to live by depends, in great part, on your personal value system. The guiding principles, however, are universal in nature. My belief is that among these universal principles are the following: Most people want to live a happy and productive life. They want to live this life free to make sound decisions for themselves, their loved ones, and their communities, and most of us want to live as long and as healthily as possible. The following are my rules for maintaining a healthy body, and consequently, healthy eyes:

1. With the help of a nutritionist, if necessary, devise an eating plan that reflects the new standards set by the United States Healthful Food Council. A plan that includes the essential food groups and a moderate exercise routine designed for you is a winning plan.
2. Avoid using caffeine and alcohol; they can often be detrimental to overall health and of the retina in particular.
3. Eliminate sodas and other caffeinated and carbonated drinks.

4. Excessive use of alcohol causes severe problems to the body, mind, and spirit, and it often causes irreparable damage to the eyes.

5. Avoid dependency on drugs, including the excessive use of prescription drugs. Drug use and dependency continues to be prevalent in the United States. With certain drugs, an accelerated deterioration is entirely possible if left unchecked. Physical, mental, and emotional deterioration are detrimental to the body, mind, and spirit. Long-term use of drugs, including some prescribed drugs, may be damaging to your eyes. Make sure to consult a doctor about the effects of drugs on the eyes and the retina.

6. Manmade fats, such as corn oil and safflower oil, as well as vegetable oils, such as canola oil and margarine, should be used in moderation or not at all. I have opted to use olive oil in general or no oil at all in many cases. Not only will you physically feel better by making these changes, but you will also propagate good healthy retinas.

7. It is wise to read about trans fats—hydrogenated vegetable oils—for your edification. There are "good" fats and "bad" fats. I made sure I knew which was which.

8. Stop eating foods that are deep-fried, overly salty, and full of monosodium glutamate. These are all toxic substances for your retina. In particular, many foods do not need additional salt. Too much salt is detrimental to your blood pressure, and high blood pressure can affect your vision.

9. Avoid the excessive consumption of sugar. Once again, it is wise to read the latest research on different types of sugars and to learn how they affect the body. Your health depends on how knowledgeable you become.

10. Do research with help from a nutritionist about a good multivitamin designed for eye health.

11. Drink a lot of water. I try to drink forty or more glasses a day,

12. Stop smoking. This produces toxic substances that affect your whole body—especially your eyes. Nicotine can rob your eyes of needed oxygen.

13. Be knowledgeable about the medications you've been prescribed and how they may affect your eyes. Consult your doctor anytime you notice a shift in your vision while on a medication.

14. Pay attention to your inner self. Stress has a way of adversely affecting the whole body and your psyche. It is important to counteract and manage the stress in our lives and the daily battering of our senses. Staying healthy encompasses knowing what causes us stress and finding ways to deal with it. Whether the stress is environmental or psychological, we have to stay physically and mentally healthy. Exercise, reading/writing (use alternative aids if needed), meditation, music/art therapy, counseling, social interaction, and nurturing, loving, supportive relationships are all ways of dealing with physical and emotional stress. For the more adventuresome among us, the sky is literally the limit (skydiving comes to mind).

15. Rest your eyes. Many Cone Rod Dystrophy patients with residual vision are working and using some bit of vision in their daily lives. Such is my case. The strain this places on the eyes, and therefore the body, can be debilitating. I found that I needed to retreat to cool dark places to reenergize. Don't fight the feeling; your eyes need to rest from daily tasks. For those who no longer have residual vision or are completely blind, winding down and resting your mind is essential.

16. Find faith. To sustain the mind and the spirit, and thereby promote a feeling of well being is a healing power; most of us find something in which we can believe. Whether one practices a religion, observes cultural practices, cultivates value systems, follows beliefs, routines, or habits, or other faith/spiritually based circumstances, what matters is finding that which nourishes

your spirit. Others find comfort, depth, and meaning in other ways. To the extent that these are positive influences in your life, you can find comfort and meaning in the things that happen to you. I found that faith helps me, and those in my life, to come to terms with my eye condition. Today, the facts of my going blind and my ability to keep faith are both sources of my inspiration, courage, and overall healing power.

CHAPTER 12:
THE AMERICANS WITH DISABILITIES ACT (ADA)

A brief understanding of the Americans with Disabilities Act (ADA) and the provisions for individuals with vision loss

Becoming disabled under any circumstances, whether it is a temporary or permanent disability, is a traumatic experience. It is hoped that wherever a disabled individual resides, there will be disability services available. It is through such services, combined with opportunities for rehabilitation, that disabled individuals can find hope.

In my native country, the Dominican Republic, there are very few services available, especially in small towns. Today, disability services in the country are provided primarily by charitable organizations and private centers. There are some international programs that provide disability services to communities. Those who have access to funds, whether from sources such as these or through family members, fare much better in managing their disabilities. The future is bleak for the vast majority who are poor. Most disabled people are cared for in family members' homes. Many families take good care of their disabled kin, offering them whatever support they can give relative to their economic status.

In these households, the disabled person are fed, clothed, and schooled at least in basic personal care. Some of these individuals may even do small chores or learn some kind of work. This care does not supplant what a center or agency can do, but it does ensure that these disabled persons are not relegated to the streets to fend for themselves—a situation that often leads to abuse of the individual. Many are simply left to beg or die. Sadly, some households are rampant with abuse and neglect.

In such households, ill treatment, such as malnutrition, lack of hygienic and medical care, and terrible physical and mental abuse is more likely to be the norm. Basic rights are routinely ignored. It is common in such situations for the disabled individual to be forced to live in the worst areas of the house or even in the backyard in makeshift housing. I have witnessed firsthand the kind of verbal abuse and cruel treatment heaped on disabled family members. I have also been witness to the great love and attention with which others surround their loved ones.

A very good friend in my hometown has a daughter who was born with Down syndrome. I have much respect and admiration for her because she fought against her family to keep her daughter. Family members wanted to institutionalize her daughter when she was a little girl. My friend courageously turned her back on the family members who offered no other support to her or the baby. Her daughter is now fifteen years old. The years of raising her daughter have not been easy, and they have taken their toll in many ways. Yet, against all odds, my friend has managed to raise her daughter in a truly admirable way. These stories are rare, but they do exist.

In the United States, as a contrast, a comprehensive civil rights act was made law in 1990. This law protects the rights of people who are challenged in any number of ways. This civil rights act is the Americans with Disabilities Act. Similar to the discrimination prohibitions in the Civil Rights Act of 1964, this law prohibits discrimination based on disability, which, as defined in the law, is given broad scope and detail. Fundamentally, the law states that a disability may be physical, mental, or emotional in nature. The law further states that the disability qualitatively limits the ability of a person to carry on with regular tasks in daily living. If the disability affects major life activities, the disabled individual has protection under the law.

The disabled individual is entitled to fairness in employment, access to adequate public/private accommodations, accessibility to public/private spaces and places, and access to activities sponsored by local, state, and federal entities. On an ongoing basis, the law is updated to include new ways to uphold the rights of the disabled individual. In addition to the aforementioned services, disabled persons are also entitled to access to transportation services, and recently, access to telecommunications systems. In the era of wide use of the Internet, groups and organizations are lobbying to expand the law to take into account the need for Internet access.

The law offers protections for disabled workers against discrimination in the workplace. If the disabled worker is qualified to do the job, he or she is not to be deterred from applying for a position within his or her qualifications. Deterrents can take place at any point in the job-seeking process, but the law is clear. Disabled workers are to be dealt with fairly during the interview and selection process. Finally, if hired, the disabled person should be given reasonable accommodations in the workplace.

Although criticisms against particular parts of the law exist, it remains the best protection to date for people with disabilities. One of the most frequently voiced criticisms is the objection to some of the language used in the law, namely the words *disabled* and *disabilities*. Similar to the now largely discarded use of *handicap* and *handicapped*, critics view the words *disabled* and *disability* as derogatory and a detriment to promoting a more positive view and perception of differently abled individuals.

One of my friends involved with lobbying efforts is fond of stating that she is "in no way broken or malfunctioning." She and the majority of disabled people consider themselves whole and essential contributing members of society. Some argue that the term denotes the inability of a person to take care of herself in daily tasks, work, having a family, and any of the great number of life achievements that are the hallmarks of independence.

On the other side of the discourse, there are those who argue that individuals with conditions that impede major life activities are indeed incapable of doing these tasks independently. These well-meaning folks prefer the law to take on a more protectionist tone. They are convinced that the disabled should be taken care of within their families, through organizations in centers, or in institutions. Those who expound these views are motivated by the desire to assuage their conscience and to alleviate the taxpayers' burden.

Whatever the motivations on either side of the question, what is fundamental to the debate is to understand the law and its purpose. Individuals who are challenged in ways described in the law are still deserving of a quality of life that allows them to live as independently as possible. They should be viewed with respect, and they should be given the same dignity that all human beings deserve to receive. This can be achieved if we are to view the Americans with Disabilities Act as a fluid document that allows for flexibility and change as people and society change. The future will bring new technologies, research, treatments, and cures for many disabling conditions. The laws in place to protect the civil rights of disabled individuals should be flexible enough to incorporate these future realities.

The debate will continue for years to come. Are disabled persons capable of living independently, and can they continue to be integrated into society? Or, are they to be taken care of and protected, and remain semi-dependent? No doubt, the debate will continue to generate passion and conflict, but ideas and resolutions will be born out of the debate. The spectrum of ideas will fine-tune and improve the law in the years to come. The law should continue to protect the evolution of future abilities that disabled people may acquire by new technologies, while at the same time avoid the erosion of the hard fought and hard won rights enshrined in the Americans with Disabilities Act.

In 2010, we celebrated the twentieth anniversary of the passage of the Americans with Disabilities Act. There were many activities in Washington DC to commemorate the occasion. I happened to catch a panel discussion on a cable television program regarding how the bill came about, the legislators that were instrumental in supporting the legislation, and the groups, organizations, and individuals that were involved in its drafting.

A lively part of the discussion was on the topic of what still needs to be done. One interesting debate among the panelists had to do with the language used in the act. The consensus was that the current language had been used to ensure passage of the bill. Yet that same language can often be a hindrance to real progress for the disabled. Among the questionable language was the use of the terms *special education, reasonable accommodations*, and *independence*.

In the case of special education, today's activists feel that this designation works to isolate and differentiate among the disabled. They feel the term promotes the attitude among some in society that the disabled person is somehow different, feeble, feebleminded, and dependent. The term *reasonable accommodations* leaves employers and others with vague impressions of what they should or should not be doing to assist the disabled. It is left to interpretation; what is reasonable to one person connotes something entirely different to another. The greatest interchange among these panelists was surrounding the concepts of individuality and independence.

The question becomes how these ideas are conceptualized and characterized by others relative to disabled persons, and to blind people in particular. An individual who happens to be blind is no different fundamentally from others. Personality characteristics continue to form along the normal developmental continuum for children and adults whether they are blind or sighted. Just as with any life-changing event, one will go through many stages when vision loss occurs, including the overwhelming shock of the diagnosis and the full significance of the prognosis.

Patients with Cone Rod Dystrophy may go through a period of denial, distress, and even depression when they learn that there is no cure for the condition. As the individual adjusts to and copes with the demands of life as a blind person, she learns that acceptance of her condition and willingness to learn the skills necessary for living will give her a more positive outlook. The ability to achieve this movement towards managing life as a blind person is in part dependent on what kind of person you are. It also takes into consideration the support systems you have in your life and the quality of the professional services and resources you have access to.

Adjusting to one's blindness is also a measure of how one feels about the blind. If our outlook is that blind people should be respected for their individualism and encouraged to be as self-reliant, self-sufficient, and as independent as possible, this will bode well for the acceptance of one's own blindness. Better adjustment will be achieved when the individual is in a positive place regarding feelings and attitudes towards the blind and being blind.

I recall when my children were small and had the can-do attitude that is so typical of children. My son was adamant about learning to ride a bike. As all children do, he wanted me to be by his side as he learned to pedal, took his falls, got up, and got on his bike again. He wanted to have me there to encourage and support him when he was failing to stay on his bike, yet give him the freedom to do it by himself.

My daughter was our family social director. She was a constant fountain of new ideas for the entire family to get involved in. She would write plays for our family to all act in, direct us all, and act in them herself. She did not want any help from anyone, but we had to cooperate. Yet, invariably, the moment would come when she was uncertain about something with the play and would come to me for advice. I had to wait her out, and I still do, but if she needs help, she asks for it. However, to this day, as an adult, my daughter embraces her can-do attitude.

I see the same pattern in my granddaughter today. She often says, "I can do it, tita," or "No, tita, it is my turn." To my feisty angel, whom I call "cookie face," I must say, "Yes you can, but just let me know if you need my help!" And of course, the time comes when she does.

Adjusting to going blind is similarly a liberal mixture of the need for independence and self-sufficiency; yet, one must recognize moments when one must depend on others for assistance. Those around us aid us best when they can distinguish between the times we need help and those when we are best left to figure it out. It is up to us to help others recognize the difference. In fact, it is up to us to help them fathom that we are actually interdependent.

The sighted are well aware of this interdependency. Young mothers may join a carpool because they realize that this method works very well when children are involved in sports, music, and other extracurricular activities. It is humanly impossible to be in all places at all times. This dependency on other mothers to help in car-pooling children around ought not to reflect poorly on the mother. Sharing tasks makes sense. Similarly, a blind person needing to have a reader to help him complete a task ought not to undermine the independence of the individual.

Others are best able to assist us when they recognize that there are times when help is needed and know when it is time to encourage and support the fledgling efforts of the blind individual. If the visually disabled person is unrealistically independent, he may place himself or others in risky or adverse situations, whereas dependent individuals are stagnant in their efforts to move forward with confidence. The danger is that they will never become self-sufficient. The key to a happier life is to learn the things you need to do on your own, and recognize when you need assistance.

The most important argument for practicing inter-dependence is how it affects your self-esteem. Being independent and self-sufficient can make you feel confident, motivated, and positive about the future. This helps you feel good about yourself and your accomplishments. Yet, trying repeatedly to do something that is outside of your capacity has the opposite effect. Asking for aid is not a sign of weakness; rather, it demonstrates the intelligence of recognizing your options. The result is the same; you move forward. Thus, the measure of how the blind individual achieves this goal is rooted in what personality traits, inner strength, support systems, organizational assistance, and resources are available to them. Certainly, being independent and self-sufficient is the ultimate goal, and getting there is the intelligent choice.

It thus becomes very important for the blind individual to have access to all of these components, because a self-sufficient, productive individual experiences heightened self-esteem and is thus better able to contribute to society.

For all these reasons, the Americans with Disabilities Act is a fluid document that is continually being improved so that Americans who are disabled can continue to move from dependency to self-sufficiency.

Blindness is not an excuse to become someone other than who we are. The visually impaired person continues being the same person with the same desires for retaining his or her individualism and feelings of independence. These elements contribute to the person's overall sense of well-being and happiness.

CHAPTER 13:
THE AFFORDABLE HEALTH CARE
FOR AMERICA ACT OF 2009

A brief understanding of the Affordable Health Care
for America Act of 2009 and how it can
help individuals with vision loss

President Barack Obama signed the Affordable Health Care for America Act into law in 2009. For the first time in the history of the United States, all American citizens have access to quality, stable, secure, affordable, and portable health care. The act makes health care more accessible, primarily due to the insurance reforms that have been brought into effect.

The Affordable Health Care for America Act embodies President Obama's most important principles for health care reform. The law works to slow down the growth of escalating health care costs; bans discrimination by insurers based on pre-existing conditions, poverty, gender, or other extrinsic discriminatory factors; establishes a market place to spur competition to keep health care affordable and portable; it promotes honesty among insurers, protects patient's rights, specifically, their choice of providers, doctors, and health care plans. Finally, it makes sure all Americans have a means of gaining access to health care through subsidies for those who do not have the funds to pay for healthcare and by allowing young adults to stay on their parents' health insurance plan longer.

Disabled Americans are blanketed as well by the healthcare act's regulations. No longer are the poorest disabled individuals forced to receive care solely from charitable organizations, non-profits, and government entities. Research shows that the disadvantaged are more prone to serious and terminal illnesses because of the lack of information, education, accessibility, and affordability to quality, stable health care. The research makes clear that those who have access to better health care are healthier and live longer.

In fact, for those who may have a job that provides them with adequate care, there are carefully considered mechanisms to improve their health care options. Foremost among these options is that the bill will keep their health care costs from escalating dramatically. The problem of staying healthy has been shamefully woeful for the uninsured, low income, the disabled, and the poor. For those who do not receive health care through an employer, or who may be self-employed or uninsured due to other factors, the proposed health care market exchange option will offer a low cost way to find a health care plan that meets their needs. Quite a number of disabled persons rely on Medicare and Medicaid for their care; however, many disabled persons do not qualify. The Medicare and Medicaid programs are addressed in relation to the benefits that are provided for disabled individuals who are covered by these plans. It is gratifying to know that there are options for disabled persons who are not under the umbrella of these plans.

Since the passage of the healthcare act, there have been ongoing attempts to amend it or even repeal it. Amendments to the bill are sure to continue. It is my hope that the bill is made stronger. As time goes by, it is my further hope that the amendments proposed will be of great assistance to the disabled, and in particular, the visually challenged. Currently, one amendment passed in the bill assures that there will be long-term care services, including home-based and community-based services. Every state within the United States recognizes that the population of poor and disabled individuals has increased and will continue to do so as circumstances arise in the lives of individuals and as populations grow older. Many of these people will be added to the state's Medicaid rolls.

The federal government, through the Affordable Health Care for America Act, has made a commitment to provide additional funds for amplifying the Medicaid rolls to manage services for these disabled individuals. The visually impaired are covered under these provisions as well. Not only is this commitment a moral imperative, but in the long run, this is a cost-effective option. Access to health care assists people in practicing preventative care. Prevention, in turn, provides for a healthier populace. Healthy communities and individuals are the best possible outcome for a healthier society.

Lobbying efforts have made a major impact in regards to the needs of blind and visually impaired individuals as they relate to the health care act. Lobbying by organizations that offer support to this population has provided guidance to legislators as they've established the framework for the bill. Specific language has been added to different parts of the bill to strengthen the existing language in the Americans with Disabilities Act (ADA).

There has been a concerted effort to assure that the health care act be aligned as much as possible to the Americans with Disabilities Act. Any changes to the bill must adhere to certain core principles for the care of the disabled.

Disabilities are natural occurrences that may affect anyone. The denial of pre-existing conditions is banned by the Affordable Health Care for America Act, as is discrimination based on disabilities. As in many populations, the disabled are quite often disabled through no act of their own. Therefore, the health care options should be seen as a continuum that reflects what all people need. Everyone needs accessibility, affordability, portability, quality, and stability in the health care plans available to them. In the interest of a healthy society, all those who are uninsured need these options as well.

This is also the case for many of the disabled who will need help through state plans or community-based organizations to receive the care they need. People with disabilities, and in particular, those with vision loss and those who do not have health care coverage will now have help in finding and paying for health care. Whether it is through the health insurance exchange, subsidies, or the amplification of community clinics, those who have vision issues will be able to find a program to meet their needs. This law makes it possible to live life as a disabled person in a meaningful, qualitative, respectful, and dignified way in conjunction with already existing services through the Americans with Disabilities Act, and through state and federal government assistance, community groups, and national organizations.

The bill is constructed on the premise that all Americans deserve respect and dignity concerning the issue of health care. Every disabled American must have the right to respect and dignity as he or she gets sicker or gets older. One's disability or aging related factors ought not serve as reasons for denial by health care systems. Through the Affordable Health Care for America Act, providers must assure that health care services are delivered in ways that demonstrate these core values. The true integrity of a nation and its people has often been said to depend on the extent to which the very young, the very old, and the disabled are treated. The Affordable Health Care for America Act of 2009 seems promising in its depth and breadth to address this fundamentally American way of being.

AFTERWORD

Happy journeys, happy endings, and looking forward to a bright future

I once asked a very significant person in my life if he believed in happy endings. Very diplomatically and in quintessentially masculine form, he explained, "I believe in a happy journey." I do agree with that observation. Humans tend to characterize life's journey as an essentially happy one if the majority of moments encompassing the journey have been happy ones. Whether they are long- or short-lived, these moments are there to look back on. We hope that these happy times have specific objectives. Preferably, these objectives will lead to positive outcomes. Whatever the objectives are, if we have positive outcomes, and if we feel we have fulfilled those objectives, that is a happy ending.

Unfulfilled goals, failures, and sadness are part of our human condition, and as such, they are part of this journey we call life; yet, juxtaposed to these are goals we do reach, and our happiness is derived from the achievable. Battling the challenges we face and experiencing the lows are part of our humanity. Moments of joy and the hope of triumph over those challenges is our very human reward. We strive for these moments. They allow us to bear the low points of our existence.

Learning to live with going blind due to Cone Rod Dystrophy has been my greatest challenge. At the onset of my blindness story, I thought I faced, in the words of the song "The Impossible Dream," an unbeatable foe. I have realized that beating the greatest challenge of my life has been measured by the extents to which I am willing to go. Once I came to terms with the overwhelming sadness and fear of losing my sight, what remained was a kind of clarity of mind. This clarity forced me to a call for action. I determined the steps I was willing to take to continue functioning in an effective and productive way. Taking actionable steps, setting achievable goals, reaching objectives, practicing being courageous and determined, accentuating the possible, and minimizing the impossible were just some of the steps I took to find those happy moments in my life.

Someone said it, and it is true: "If you can believe, you can achieve." I believe this wholeheartedly. Believing you can do something is the first and most dramatic step. Prioritizing, setting goals, and establishing and implementing a plan of action are necessary to accomplish what you have set out to do. Whatever model you use is up to you; just have a plan to manage your lifestyle change due to visual impairment, and you will have success. The challenges that come your way need not defeat you, unless you succumb. Rather than give up, find your way to conquer them; this will bring you greater happiness. You know that there will be challenges ahead. If you can take the incremental and necessary steps to deal with them, and if you are consistent in finding courage and support along the way, you will surprise yourself. When you do that, there will come a day when you realize that you are learning, becoming, being productive, having fun, minimizing your unhappy times, and maximizing your happy ones.

My happy journey continues as I follow through with goals I have set for myself. There undoubtedly will be challenging, distressing, and perhaps even unhappy times. I look upon these as opportunities to find the best way to make things work so that I can accomplish my goals. Although accommodation is a liberal part of my vocabulary, limitations are not. The more I learn how to manage my Cone Rod Dystrophy, the more confident, productive, secure, and happier I am.

Thus, my journey is one of discovery, life, love, and laughter, and that is what happy endings are all about.

This is what I will continue to do as long as I live. What is certain is that I will be a blind person. It is a part of my totality as an individual. Just as certain as I am of being Dominican, a citizen, a teacher, a daughter, a sister, a mother, a grandmother, a godmother, an aunt, a cousin, a colleague, a friend, and a lover—I am certain that blindness does not define me; it accentuates me.

The most critical step in my journey of discovering who I can be as a blind person began with a strong base of knowledge about my condition. Through dialogue with doctors and low vision specialists, I gained a thorough understanding of the nature of being blind, what the particular effects of my condition were for me, and the tools and strategies I would need. Working with groups, organizations, state and federal agencies, and others has been the foundation for my emotional support, and this has given me access to the current research and treatments available. It is important to stay informed of the research entities that are producing a great deal of studies pertaining to eye conditions. Knowledge will inspire confidence and motivation in your loved ones and in you. This motivation to know what new research is saying or what new treatments are becoming available is not just due to self-interest; it ought to be for the benefit of loved ones and others affected by your prognosis, such as friends and loved ones.

There are numerous resources available in the United States to assist an individual with blindness and visual impairments. Become skillful at searching the Internet. Seek out people who are affected so you can support one another in tremendous ways. Talk to doctors and other eye professionals on an ongoing basis in order to keep up a good, healthy regimen for your body, mind, and spirit. Work on establishing trusting, honest relationships that you have taken the time to nurture. These relationships will provide the impetus you need to bravely move forward to meet and surpass each challenge. Strengthened by knowledge, armed with new skills, and moving forward with renewed confidence, you will be able to meet the future with optimism. At the same time, you will help others around you learn more about your condition and how they can best be of assistance to you.

Included here are some of the more prevalent and well-known organizations doing research and working to help individuals affected by eye conditions. It is my hope that this book will help on this leg of the journey. It is overwhelming at first to try to absorb everything you need to know all at once. I had to set a reasonable pace for myself. Only you will know what you need to learn, and when you need to learn it.

I often think back to when I was reading all those baby books to find out if my babies were reaching the suggested benchmarks at the "right" age. Like everyone else, I read the chapters I needed to read as the child reached a particular milestone. There is a reason why such benchmarks are grouped chronologically. Parents can become overwhelmed by the immensity of information directed toward them. Parents only want to focus on what they need to know for their child at a particular age or stage of development.

Expect that some of the information you learn may pertain to your particular eye condition and some may not. Realize that certain descriptors will readily refer to your situation, but recognize that many conditions mimic each other. Eye doctors and professionals will help make this information relevant for you. Be aware that some of what you will learn may affect you emotionally. You may feel sad, hopeless, or depressed by what you learn. These feelings are only natural and normal, given the circumstances. I have learned that this is part of the grieving process. Losing your sight is like losing a loved one. There are mental health professionals, counseling groups, and organizations ready to help you overcome these challenges. They can help you adjust to the loss of your vision, and they can help make that loss more understandable and bearable.

Above all, practice bravery and keep faith. Happier times are ahead. There is hope of a happy journey for you and a happy ending as well.

A BRIEF BIBLIOGRAPHY

The following is a list of resources whose material I utilized in the writing of this book. Although this is a very brief bibliography of the resources available regarding visual disorders, they represent first-contact places for help.

Affordable Health Care for America Act
American Council of the Blind
Americans with Disabilities Act
American Foundation for the Blind
Doheny Eye Institute
Foundation Fighting Blindness
Georgetown Center for Sight
International Council for Education of People with Visual Impairments
Lighthouse International
Lions Club
Mobility International
National Association of Blind Students
National Association for Visually Handicapped
National Association for Parents of Children with Visual Impairments
National Eye Institute at National Institutes of Health
National Federation of the Blind
National Library Service for the Blind and Physically Handicapped
Prevent Blindness America

Recordings for the Blind and Dyslexic
Sensory Access Foundation
The Knights Templar Eye Foundation
The World Health Organization
University of Michigan Kellogg Eye Center
Vision Foundation, Inc.
Vision World Wide
Wilmer Eye Institute at Johns Hopkins
*You may also contact your state's department for the blind and visually impaired.

** If I left out any source on my resource list, please contact me at:
vida.byas@yahoo.com

www.ingramcontent.com/pod-product-compliance
Lightning Source LLC
Chambersburg PA
CBHW070018300526
45794CB00001B/353